"With topics ranging from vaccination hesitancy to wellness influencers, this edited volume provides a timely and nuanced approach to understand the current crisis of public trust in biomedical expert knowledge. Throughout the book, pioneering research tackles the socio-cultural dynamics at the core of this phenomenon, but it also highlights the importance of collaborating across different academic disciplines, as well as beyond academia, with journalists and debunkers. As increased awareness and critical knowledge of the harmful consequences of non-scientific health practices become more and more urgent, this book is a most informative starting point for researchers, policy makers and the general public alike."

—Dr Maria Vaccarella, Lecturer in Medical Humanities, University of Bristol, UK

"Medical Misinformation and Social Harm in Non-Science-Based Health Practices *is a highly readable and original collection inviting the readers to embark on their own intellectual journey into the impressive array of disciplines it touches upon and very skilfully synthesises: criminology, digital sociology, health psychology, medicine, law, investigative journalism and even quantum physics! A thought-provoking, relevant and important work that needs to be read."*

—Professor Georgios A. Antonopoulos, Professor of Criminology, Teesside University, UK

"There have been several excellent critical analyses of non-science-based healthcare in recent years. This book, a multi-author, multi-disciplinary investigation into bogus health practices and claims, is amongst the best in this tradition. The authors look at the subject from refreshingly different perspectives including criminology, health fraud, quantum woo, pseudoscience, science denial, nutritional fads, fake herbal medicine, anti-vaccination rhetoric, and journalism. They provide important critical analyses that complement each other and provide a fully rounded picture.

Non-science-based health practices cause untold psychological, physical, and economic damage to consumers, patients and society. This scholarly volume will help us to better understand the often-complex issues involved. I recommend it to all who wish to minimise the dangers of misinformation in medicine."

—Professor Edzard Ernst, Emeritus Professor, University of Exeter, UK. Former Professor in Physical Medicine and Rehabilitation and Chair in Complementary Medicine

"In this original and timely collection, Lavorgna and Di Ronco gather a range of experts from across disciplines to expose the complex harms associated with non-science-based health practices. In an age of creeping healthcare privatisation, patient-consumer sovereignty, online networking and e-commerce, this book brings much-needed refinement to current conversations about pseudoscience and quackery. Cutting-edge social science at its best, this book will be of interest not only to students and academics in criminology, sociology, health and law, but also to practitioners and policy makers working to protect the public from fraudulent medical practices and health misinformation."

—Dr Alexandra Hall, Senior Lecturer in Criminology, Northumbria University, UK

Medical Misinformation and Social Harm in Non-Science-Based Health Practices

Fraudulent, harmful, or at best useless pharmaceutical and therapeutic approaches developed outside science-based medicine have boomed in recent years, especially due to the commercialisation of cyberspace. The latter has played a fundamental role in the rise of false 'health experts', and in the creation of filter bubbles and echo chambers that have contributed to the formation of highly polarised debates on non-science-based health practices—online as well as offline.

By adopting a multidisciplinary approach, this edited book brings together contributions of international academics and practitioners from criminology, digital sociology, health psychology, medicine, law, physics, and journalism, where they critically analyse different types of non-science-based health approaches. With this volume, we aim to reconcile different scientific understandings of these practices, synthesising a variety of empirical, theoretical and interpretative approaches, and exploring the challenges, implications and potential remedies to the spread of dangerous and misleading health information.

This edited book will offer some food for thought not only to students and academics in the social sciences, health psychology and medicine among other disciplines, but also to medical practitioners, science journalists, debunkers, policy makers and the general public, as they might all benefit from a greater awareness and critical knowledge of the harms caused by non-scientific health practices.

Anita Lavorgna, PhD, is Associate Professor in Criminology at the University of Southampton. She is currently leading research projects on internet-facilitated wildlife trafficking and harmful alternative health practices. Anita's research pivots around cybercrimes (especially trafficking activities online), serious and organised crime, and the propagation of misleading and fraudulent health information.

Anna Di Ronco, PhD, is Senior Lecturer in Criminology at the Sociology Department of the University of Essex. Her research interests lie in the regulation, representation, and enforcement of incivilities regulations, and individuals' resistance to social control in the physical and digital space. Her more recent projects look into the local collaborative governance of prostitution in European cities and into the role of social media in supporting (otherwise criminalised or silenced) environmental activism.

Routledge Studies in Crime and Society

Execution by Family
A Theory of Honor Violence
Mark Cooney

Changing Narratives of Youth Crime
From Social Causes to Threats to the Social
Bernd Dollinger

Human Enhancement Drugs
Edited by Katinka van de Ven, Kyle J.D. Mulrooney and Jim McVeigh

Organized Crime and Terrorist Networks
Edited by Vincenzo Ruggiero

Private Security and Domestic Violence
The Risks and Benefits of Private Security Companies Working with Victims of Domestic Violence
Diarmaid Harkin

The Human Factor of Cybercrime
Edited by Rutger Leukfeldt and Thomas J. Holt

Medical Misinformation and Social Harm in Non-Science-Based Health Practices
A Multidisciplinary Perspective
Edited by Anita Lavorgna and Anna Di Ronco

For more information about this series, please visit: www.routledge.com/Routledge-Studies-in-Crime-and-Society/book-series/RSCS

Medical Misinformation and Social Harm in Non-Science-Based Health Practices

A Multidisciplinary Perspective

Edited by Anita Lavorgna and Anna Di Ronco

Routledge
Taylor & Francis Group
LONDON AND NEW YORK

First published 2020
by Routledge
2 Park Square, Milton Park, Abingdon, Oxon OX14 4RN

and by Routledge
52 Vanderbilt Avenue, New York, NY 10017

Routledge is an imprint of the Taylor & Francis Group, an informa business

First issued in paperback 2021

British Library Cataloguing-in-Publication Data
A catalogue record for this book is available from the British Library

Library of Congress Cataloging-in-Publication Data
A catalog record has been requested for this book

ISBN: 978-1-138-38866-6 (hbk)
ISBN: 978-1-03-208753-5 (pbk)
ISBN: 978-0-429-42443-4 (ebk)

Typeset in Bembo
by Apex CoVantage, LLC

To Leonardo—may you grow up in a world that is wiser and healthier for all

Anita

To my mother, Marta, Jacqueline, Giorgia, and all New Year's Eve little boats, which gave me food for thought for this book

Anna

Contents

Figures

Tables

Figures

Tables

Contributors

James Allen-Robertson is Lecturer in Media and Communication and Computational Sociologist in the Department of Sociology at the University of Essex. Dr Allen-Robertson's early book *Digital Culture Industry* (2013) charted the role of piracy in the development of digital media distribution. His more recent work explores issues of power and agency in the relationship between humans and their media machines and seeks to develop new computational methods for social science research.

Craig A. Anderson is Distinguished Professor of Psychology, Iowa State University. His early work focused on attribution theory and social judgment processes. His current work focuses on the General Aggression Model, a bio-social-cognitive model integrating aggression theories from social, personality, developmental, and cognitive psychology. Much of his recent empirical work involves media effects. In 2017, Dr Anderson received the Kurt Lewin Award from the Society for the Psychological Study of Psychological Issues, for 'outstanding contributions to the development and integration of psychological research and social action.' In 2018, he received the Society for Personality and Social Psychology's Distinguished Scholar Award.

David Barron is Deputy Director and Senior Research Fellow at the Perdana University Centre for Psychological Medicine. Dr Barron has been actively involved in research related to psychology, especially with personality, and has published extensively in numerous acclaimed international journals.

Felicity L. Bishop is a registered Health Psychologist and Associate Professor at the University of Southampton. Dr Bishop's research focuses on patients' beliefs and decision-making about treatment. She has published widely on how and why patients utilise complementary and alternative medicines, the psychosocial factors and processes that contribute to the effects of complementary and alternative medicines (particularly in musculoskeletal disorders), and patients' experiences of and views on placebo effects. She is particularly interested in developing and testing ethical ways to enhance placebo effects in clinical practice.

Emilie Cloatre is Professor of Law at Kent Law School, and Principal Investigator for the Wellcome Trust project 'Law, Medicines and "Modern Healthcare": Regulating Traditional and Alternative Medicines in Contemporary Contexts'. Her publications include *Pills for the Poorest: An Exploration of TRIPS and Access to Medication in Africa* (2013) and *Knowledge, Technology and Law* (2014, Routledge).

Ilario D'Amato is a journalist and the author of *Dossier Hamer* (2017), a book resulting from a 10-year-long inquiry into the fraudulent anti-cancer ideas promoted by the Germanic New Medicine system. After graduating from the University of Salerno in 2011 with a bachelor's degree in communication sciences, he earned a master's degree in international journalism from City, University of London in 2013 and a master's in communication for development from the University of Malmö in 2017. He has been multimedia editor for The Climate Group and is now digital manager for The Royal Star & Garter Homes.

Enrico Gazzola obtained his PhD in Physics in 2014 at the University of Padova. Dr Gazzola's post-doctoral research activities mainly focused on the of applications of nano-optics to biosensors and of structured light to telecommunications. More recently, he moved to nuclear physics topics, related to neutron detection. He is devoted to science dissemination, especially about quantum physics and the problems of pseudoscience, through conferences, social networks, and his book *Il mondo quantistico* ['The Quantum World'] (2017).

Heather Horsburgh is Teaching Fellow in Criminology at the University of Southampton. Dr Horsburgh's research interests lie within criminology and psychology and include media and criminal justice, occupational health of emergency services, and information sharing and accountability in criminal justice, political, and health spheres.

Ganna Isayeva is Head of the Department of Complex Risk Reduction of Chronic Non-communicable Diseases, National Institute of Therapy in Ukraine. Dr Isayeva graduated from Kharkiv National University in 1998 in Ukraine and completed her PhD in preventive cardiology in 2004. She specialises in lipidology, hypertension disease, and diabetes mellitus. She is the author of more than 100 publications in preventive medicine.

Rosa Koenraadt is Lecturer in Criminology at the Institute of Criminal Law and Criminology, Leiden University, the Netherlands. Dr Koenraadt conducts research in the area of cultural criminology, illegal markets, and human trafficking.

Anna Markovska is Principal Lecturer in Criminology, School of Humanities and Social Sciences, Anglia Ruskin University. Dr Markovska has written widely on the issues of corruption and organised crime in Ukraine. She has recently been involved in three educational projects sponsored by the British Council in Ukraine and was the recipient of British Academy grants to study migration, policing, and corruption.

Ester Massa is Lecturer in Criminology at the University of Winchester. Dr Massa holds a specific expertise on quantitative research, focusing on multiple topics such as juvenile delinquency, immigration and criminalisation processes, prisonisation, and gender differences in the criminal justice system.

Sergyi Ostropolets is Senior Lecturer in Medical Informatics at the VN Karazin Kharkiv National University School of Medicine. He has an MA in biomedical systems engineering from Kharkiv National University of Radio Electronics. He subsequently completed post-graduate courses (mathematical modeling and numerical analysis in medical research) at the VN Karazin Kharkiv National University. His research interests focus on medical data acquisition, processing, storage, and management.

Sara Prot, PhD Iowa State University 2015, is Lecturer in Social Psychology at Coventry University and Research Associate at the Centre for Advances in Behavioural Science at Coventry University. Dr Prot's research expertise is in social psychology, with an emphasis on processes underlying science denial, aggressive behaviour, prosocial behaviour, and intergroup conflict.

Nayeli Urquiza-Haas is a Wellcome Trust Research Associate at Kent University for the project 'Law, Medicines and "Modern Healthcare": Regulating Traditional and Alternative Medicines in Contemporary Contexts'. Dr Urquiza-Haas's areas of expertise include drug regulation, criminal law, and feminist legal studies.

Acknowledgements

Editing this book has been an exciting and rewarding journey, which has given us the precious opportunity to continue, or in some cases to start, a dialogue with our passionate and dedicated contributors. Our first thank you, therefore, goes to them, for getting involved and believing in this project in the first place.

We would also like to acknowledge with gratitude the participants of the final workshop of the project 'Hush the quacks. Exploring health fraud scams in the UK' held in September 2017 at the University of Southampton, and of the panel 'Endangering public health: a criminological perspective' held during the 2017 Annual Conference of the European Society of Criminology. We have learnt a lot from the discussions we had during these events, which were of inspiration and motivation in the writing and editing of this volume.

A special thank you goes to Robin West and Heather Horsburgh, for their help in proofreading some parts of this book. You are truly wonderful colleagues!

To Gianluca, from Anita: I probably would have never started to look into the dangers of certain non-science-based health practices in an academic fashion if it was not for the insightful, often intricate, and at times difficult discussions we had along the years on this topic. As always, you helped me to look deeper and wider.

1 Introduction

Anita Lavorgna and Anna Di Ronco

Why a book on non-science-based health practices, and why now?

Measles is a highly contagious viral illness affecting millions of people every year, especially in Asia and Africa. It can lead to severe complications and—in the most serious cases—even to death. Luckily, since the 1960s measles is vaccine-preventable, and over the years measles' vaccination rates have been high enough to render this disease relatively uncommon in many countries. Over the last few years, however, global vaccination rates have generally declined, and the number of measles cases has started to rise again. Preliminary global data from the World Health Organization shows that reported measles cases have increased steadily from 2017, rising to 300% in the first three months of 2019 (compared to the same period in the previous year) (WHO 2019). While in some (non-western) countries the decline in vaccination rates is linked to conflicts and supply problems, in many countries it is associated with an increased hesitance towards vaccination among those who refuse to get immunised against various diseases, including measles. Rising clusters of unvaccinated people are often linked to the spread of anti-vaccine scaremongering and misinformation suggesting that vaccinations, especially during early childhood, can cause severe reactions and even conditions such as autism. These unfounded safety concerns have gained traction over the past few years, especially due to worried parents, fake experts, and cynical public figures (such as populist politicians) trying to please their audience or attract potential voters.

The year 2019 has been an *annus horribilis* not only in relation to the decline in vaccination rates. On a daily basis, media news constantly reminds us that the erosion of trust and legitimacy of science and, more generally, of experts is still very much alive and present, as it permeates public debates—being they on climate change, the management of migration flows, or public health interventions. The consequences are not only daunting, as when it comes to health-related issues, but also often tangible and immediate. Consider, for instance, the case of Germana Durando, an Italian family doctor and 'homeopath' who, together with her mentor, Spanish physician Maria Gloria Alcover, persuaded a woman not to take evidence-based medicine to cure her skin cancer. The woman was persuaded to rely instead on alternative approaches (which led to her death in 2015) based on the dangerous and unproven ideas of Hamer, a German ex-physician. Only in late 2018 and early 2019 were the two practitioners respectively convicted of manslaughter and banned from the medical profession—something only made possible by proving the case of the victim's mental manipulation via a documented email exchange (which is usually missing, since most practitioners advocating similar quack treatments tend to be more careful about leaving a paper trail) (D'Amato 2017a, b; *La Stampa* 2019).

Other cases of potentially dangerous health-related behaviours might seem less extreme, but they can end up being equally life threatening, or otherwise have a detrimental impact of people's wellbeing. Think, for example, of the extreme eating or wellness practices adopted by some people (often encouraged by fitness bloggers and wellness 'experts'), or their thoughtless consumption of self-prescribed pharmaceuticals and supplements without proper medical supervision (Rousseau 2015; Lavorgna and Sugiura 2018; González-Stuart and Rivera 2019). Many of these dietary regimes or tablets might offer a quick fix towards an aspirational body or lifestyle, often by claiming that they are safe and 'natural'; it goes without saying that they can also cause serious harm to both mental and physical health.

In this edited book, you will encounter many cases similar to those exemplified above. They are very different in nature but are nonetheless grouped together as they all share a key, fundamental feature: they are all characterised by the fact that harm—or, better, different types of harm—has been caused to people by the use and the propagation of health practices that are not based on scientific evidence yet are nonetheless accepted or even applauded by many based on the medical misinformation received.

Fraudulent, harmful, or at best useless medical and therapeutic practices are not new. Despite the consensus in the medical discipline that certain approaches lack scientific evidence and are worthless, the promotion and selling of fake cures and wellbeing approaches advertised as safe and effective have long plagued healthcare systems, often preying on those more vulnerable (Lerner 1984; Herbert 1986; Offit 2013; Cattaneo and Corbellini 2014). Medical misinformation and non-science-based health practices, however, have boomed in recent years: the Web and social media in particular have played a fundamental role in the creation of like-minded virtual communities and in the rise of false experts (Lavorgna and Di Ronco 2017; Broniatowski et al. 2018; Klawitter and Hargittai 2018; Lavorgna and Sugiura 2018). Furthermore, as public faith in the traditional authority and power of professionals has progressively diminished, it has been increasingly easy for improvised or fraudulent health specialists to exploit the (badly placed) trust of those looking for a hope or for an alternative, easier way to solve their medical and physical problems (Rojek 2017).

In this context, approaches and treatments developed outside science-based medicine are more and more the object of highly polarised debates, with 'believers' and 'sceptics' presenting arguments for or against their legitimacy and effectiveness. 'Believers' tend to advocate their freedom in choosing what they view as natural, holistic, preventive, or otherwise effective for their physical, psychological, or spiritual needs. 'Sceptics', on their part, emphasise the need to only rely on what has been adequately tested and works rather than on non-science-based treatments and approaches, which can be dangerous and greatly harmful to people's health (especially when they take the form of frauds or cult-like quackeries) as well as to society as a whole. This polarisation, however, is toxic and is causing a stagnation, rather than a progress, in the public understanding of science and the adoption of safe and healthier behaviours (Petts and Niemeyer 2004; Schmidt et al. 2018). We believe that a greater level of critical knowledge is needed not only to better understand the dynamics of the public debate as affected by health-related misinformation, but also to unpack the causes that, at various levels, make this misinformation so appealing. Our hope is that through critical knowledge, social scientists (as well as activists and civil society) can learn to engage more productively in these debates, facilitating mutual comprehension and communication and possibly improving the public's trust in science and evidence-based pharmaceuticals and treatments. This is not an easy task, but a worthwhile and compelling one that we will seek to advance in this book.

Problematising non-science-based health practices

The term 'non-science-based health practice' is a product of modern western medicine and, more pragmatically, of the establishment of scientific medical standards for the testing of manufactured drugs and experimental treatments. In practice, this means that all health-related practices that are substandard, or have not been tested against these scientific medical standards, are, by definition, non-science-based. This is not irrelevant and without consequences: the verified conformity of health-related practices and approaches to given scientific standards may have important effects, including that of impairing or limiting their circulation and availability on the market. Health-related treatments developed in disregard of, or not in full compliance with, scientific standards may be varied: while some may be seriously dangerous and harmful to people, others may be quite harmless and relatively effectless (such as many homeopathic treatments).

For other health-related practices, however, things may be less clear-cut. This is especially the case for health-related approaches developed in socio-cultural and epistemological contexts quite removed from western societies; for these, it may be quite hard to prove compliance with the expected medical standards, as these tend to be informed only on western epistemologies (Cloatre 2019). As a result, the access to the market of these health-related practices may be challenged or limited to various degrees. An illustrative example of this, which you will encounter in this book, are plant-based healing remedies traditionally used in many non-western countries. These remedies have increasingly been pushed out of the European market through its pharmacovigilance system.

In essence, definitions of, and attitudes and responses to, non-science-based health practices are shaped by socio-cultural dynamics. Similarly, the labels used to identify the providers of non-science-based or alternative health practices are context—as well as time—specific. In between the mid-16th and the 19th centuries in Italy, for example, the label 'charlatan' did not have its current negative connotation (that is, someone pretending to have knowledge or skills they have not, a 'quack'). Charlatans were professionals (a specific category of healers) and, as such, were required to submit their remedies for inspection to *protomedico* tribunals, colleges of physicians or health offices, which ensured that they complied with certain acceptable parameters before issuing a licence to sell them (Gentilcore 2006). In a way, so-called charlatans had a professional status that is somehow similar to the one under which licensed complementary and alternative medicine providers currently operate in many jurisdictions. In pan-Indian traditions, a 'guru' is an inspirational figure, a counsellor, a spiritual guide. In common parlance, the term is now used (often in a derogatory way) to indicate any expert, even a self-declared or a fraudulent one—a meaning that ends up being disrespectful for entire cultural traditions and dharmic religions.

These examples point to the context-specific character of non-science-based health practices, as well as of the labels, frames, and narratives used to define them. The boundaries of our topic of investigation, its definitions, and the responses to it are very much shaped by the socio-cultural context in consideration. This complexity has certainly informed this multi-authored and multidisciplinary project and is reflected for instance in the different working definitions used to circumscribe the issues at stake in the various chapters.

From our initial criminological take to a multidisciplinary journey

With a very few exceptions, relatively little attention has so far been paid in the social sciences, including criminology, to the topic of misleading medical information and, specifically, of non-science-based health practices. This oversight is quite surprising as criminology in particular should be very concerned with the study of these practices, if anything because some of them are leading to immense social harms—and harm is a key concept in criminology, allowing criminologists to gaze out from the narrow boundaries of criminal justice. Particularly, non-science-based health practices can cause serious repercussions both on the health of people and on their confidence in the medical profession and the scientific method (Lavorgna and Di Ronco 2018).

Through some pilot studies (Lavorgna and Di Ronco 2017, 2018; Lavorgna and Sugiura 2018), over the past few years we have attempted to apply criminological lenses to the topic of non-science-based health practices—a research path that we believe deserves to be explored much further. However, it has been clear to us from the outset that criminology alone can grasp only a limited angle of non-science-based health practices, which is a plainly and inherently transdisciplinary issue. Thanks to a collaborative mini-grant and the resulting workshop,[1] we have started a dialogue with colleagues from other disciplines and even health practitioners on the topic. Through this dialogue, the challenges and the rewards of such an endeavour have soon come to light: one the one hand, we have noticed the difficulties in finding a common ground (and sometimes even a common language!) to effectively share knowledge and progress our investigation; on the other hand, we have had a sense of the immense possibilities (both in terms of research opportunities and potential impact) that an exchange between scholars from different disciplines and practitioners can bring to the knowledge, including the possibility to identify common research gaps and needs. Furthermore, we have also soon realised that while academic research on harmful non-science-based health practices is still quite limited, some journalists and debunkers have gained substantial knowledge on this topic over time; this experience and knowledge is important and should serve scientific purposes once submitted to academic rigour and methodological knowledge.

This edited book originates from these earlier ideas, pilot studies, and ongoing conversations. By adopting a multidisciplinary approach, it brings together contributions of international academics and practitioners from criminology, digital sociology, health psychology, medicine, law, physics, and journalism, which provide critical analyses of non-science-based health approaches. With this volume, we aim to reconcile different scientific understandings of these practices, synthesising a variety of empirical, theoretical, and interpretative approaches and exploring the challenges, implications, and potential remedies to the spread of dangerous health information.

We hope this edited book will offer some food for thought not only to students and academics in the social sciences, health psychology, and medicine among other disciplines, but also to medical practitioners, science journalists, debunkers, policy makers, and the general public, as they might all benefit from a greater awareness and critical knowledge on the harms caused by non-scientific health practices and the related misinformation.

After presenting a typology of harmful health practitioners offering non-science-based treatments (Chapter 2), the book will continue by shedding some light on the intricate net of causes that can help us in explaining the success of many non-science-based health practices. We will explore the psychological processes underlying the denial of science-based medical practices (Chapter 3) and the risk perceptions of consumers of potentially dangerous lifestyle supplements (Chapter 4). We will also address the institutional context that allows certain ineffective pseudoscientific practices to thrive (Chapter 5) and the role of the political debate in generating anti-scientific positions on healthcare issues (Chapter 6), in addition to the logical fallacies distorting the scientific jargon that create a fertile ground for impostors (Chapter 7). The volume will continue with an account of the role of social media in supporting the promotion of misleading nutrition information (Chapter 8), as well as online activism against vaccines (Chapter 9). The final part of the book considers some legal and social responses to non-science-based approaches, paying particular attention to contemporary regulatory dilemmas on the criminalisation of traditional herbal medicine (Chapter 10), the responsibility of traditional media in framing the debate on non-science-based health practices (Chapter 11), and the role of investigative journalism in tackling dangerous treatments (Chapter 12).

Note

1 Lavorgna A (criminology) and Bishop FL (health psychology), project 'Hush the quacks. Exploring health fraud scams in the UK', the 2016 Strategic Interdisciplinary Research Development Fund, Faculty of Social Sciences, University of Southampton.

References

Broniatowski DA, Jamison AM, Qi S, AlKulaib L, Chen T, Benton A, Quinn SA and Dredze M (2018) Weaponized health communication: twitter bots and Russian trolls amplify the vaccine debate. *American Journal of Public Health* 108(10):1378–1384

Cattaneo E and Corbellini G (2014) Taking a stand against pseudoscience. *Nature* 510:333–335

Cloatre E (2019) Traditional medicines, law, and the (dis)ordering of temporalities. In Beynon-Jones SM and Grabham E (eds.) *Law and time*. London, UK: Routledge

D'Amato I (2017a) *Dossier Hamer: inchiesta su una tragica premessa di cura contro il cancro*. Milan: Mondadori

D'Amato I (2017b) *Germana Durando, medico 'hameriano', condannata a due anni e mezzo in primo grado*. Available at: www.dossierhamer.it/blog/germana-durando/

Gentilcore D (2006) *Medical charlatanism in early modern Italy*. Oxford, UK: Oxford University Press

González-Stuart EA and Rivera JO (2019) Herbal weight loss supplements from dubious efficacy to direct toxicity. In Watson RR and Preedy VR (eds.) *Dietary interventions in liver disease: foods, nutrients, and dietary supplements*. London: Elsevier

Herbert V (1986) Unproven (questionable) dietary and nutritional methods in cancer prevention and treatment. *Cancer* 58(S8):1930–1941

Klawitter E and Hargittai E (2018) 'I went home to Google': how user assess the credibility of online health information. In Hale TM, Chou WYS, Cotton SR and Khilnani A (eds.) *eHealth: current evidence, promises, perils and future directions*. Bingley, UK: Emerald Publishing Limited

La Stampa (2019) Tre anni di carcere al medico che curava il cancro con l'approccio olistico. Available at: www.lastampa.it/2019/04/02/cronaca/tre-anni-di-carcere-al-medico-che-curava-il-cancro-con-lapproccio-olistico-1MifQceQ1ZexDilITOd5gJ/pagina.html

Lavorgna A and Di Ronco A (2017) Fraud victims or unwary accomplices? An exploratory study of online communities supporting quack medicine. In van Duyne PC, Harvey J, Antonopoulos GA and von Lampe K (eds.) *The many faces of crime for profit and ways of tackling it*. Oisterwijk, NL: Wolf Legal Publishers

Lavorgna A and Di Ronco A (2018) Media representations of complementary and alternative medicine in the Italian press: a criminological perspective. *European Journal of Criminology* 15(4):421–441

Lavorgna A and Sugiura L (2018) Caught in a lie: the rise and fall of a respectable deviant. *Deviant Behavior* (online first)

Lerner IJ (1984) The whys of cancer quackery. *Cancer* 53:815–819

Offit P (2013) *Killing us softly: the sense and nonsense of alternative medicine*. London: Harper Collins

Petts J and Niemeyer S (2004) Health risk communication and amplification: learning from the MMR vaccination controversy. *Health, Risk & Society* 6(1):7–23

Rojek C (2017) The case of Belle Gibson, social media, and what it means for understanding leisure under digital praxis. *Annals of Leisure Research* 20(5):524–528

Rousseau S (2015) The celebrity quick-fix: when good food meets bad science. *Food, Culture & Society* 18(2):265–287

Schmidt AL, Zollo F, Scala A, Betsch C and Quattrociocchi W (2018) Polarization of the vaccination debate on Facebook. *Vaccine* 36(25):3606–3612

WHO (2019) New measles surveillance data for 2019. Available at: www.who.int/immunization/newsroom/measles-data-2019/en/

2 Towards a better criminological understanding of harmful alternative health practices

A provider typology

Anita Lavorgna and Heather Horsburgh

Introduction

The promotion of fraudulent, dangerous, or useless medical treatments is not something new: the figure of the snake-oil salesman who sells false cures to the masses is centuries old, and in recent times it is well-documented how certain individuals prey on the fears and frustrations (when the official medicine seems unable to find a cure) of the general public to promote 'quackeries' (Bashford 1911; Lerner 1984; Offit 2013; Lavorgna and Di Ronco 2017, 2018). The commercialisation of the internet and its increasingly ubiquitous presence in our lives have opened a whole new range of opportunities for fraudsters and self-proclaimed 'experts' to disseminate erroneous and potentially dangerous health-related information and to reach for potential new costumers or followers (Holmes et al. 2017; Lavorgna and Di Ronco 2017; Delgado-López and Corrales-García 2018; Lavorgna and Sugiura 2018).

So-called quackeries are not only relevant in terms of consumer protection from financial harms; they can cause severe emotive, psychological, and health harms, and even result in the death of vulnerable individuals. Suffice it to remember how many fake treatments are directed to people suffering from cancer: as already noted by Lerner (1984), a lack of confidence in the public institutions and the public panic towards 'the big C' create a fertile soil for unorthodox alternatives to surgery, radiation, and chemotherapy (described in the 'quacks'' jargon as mutilation, burning, and poisoning). Furthermore, the promotion of these fake 'alternative' treatments impairs the trust in the scientific method and, more generally, in the medical therapeutics, causing potentially long-term societal harms (Lavorgna and Di Ronco 2017)

In the academic literature, there are limited studies on providers of harmful non-science-based health practices. As we will see in the following section, existing research suggests that these under-investigated providers should not be considered as part of a homogeneous group: many seem to be knowingly misleading their patients, for what we can suppose are a range of diverse motivations, while others seem to believe in what they do and say. This chapter will propose a multi-dimensional criminological typology[1] of providers of harmful alternative health practices, which we hope can serve as a starting point to aid our understanding of the motivations behind their actions and their modus operandi, and therefore facilitate the development of prevention and intervention strategies.

Literature review

Definitional ambiguities and motivational variety: the need for a provider typology

Complementary and alternative medicine (CAM) (also known as 'integrative medicine') is an umbrella term encompassing a broad and heterogeneous range of healthcare approaches developed outside standard science-based medicine, some of which have a positive effect on patients' physical and physiological health (Ernst et al. 2001; EFCAM 2017). Besides benign types of CAMs, however, there are a number of pseudoscientific practices that can be extremely harmful. As summarised by Offit, a way to differentiate valuable complementary treatments from dangerous pseudomedicine is that the latter is recommended against helpful conventional therapies, promotes potentially harmful therapies without adequate warning, drains patients' bank accounts, and promotes magical thinking (Offit 2013:240ff).

Defining these dangerous practices, however, is not an easy task: the 'quacks' selling them often self-denominate their treatments as CAM, but many in the CAM community do not want to be associated with dangerous pseudomedicine (Lavorgna and Bishop 2017). To complicate matters even more, part of the scientific and medical community rejects all or most CAMs altogether as 'irrational approaches to medical practice' (Angell and Kassirer 1998:3) or as 'smokescreen[s] behind which enthusiasts of dubious practices try to incorporate their unproven therapies into routine health care' (Ernst 2011:21), which further hinders the possibility to isolate and investigate dangerous forms of non-science-based medicine. Furthermore, the same CAM remedy—for instance, the use of manipulative therapies—could be used, to continue with our example, as an effective way to improve general wellness and reduce stress in patients with migraines (Wells et al. 2011; Zhang et al. 2017), but it might also be used in a very dangerous way. One example among many concerns the fake Australian chiropractor George Zaphir, who was successfully prosecuted by the Australian Health Practitioner Regulation Agency (AHPRA) in 2018 for his unlawful use of the protected title 'chiropractor' and holding out as a registered health practitioner, while stating that he had an 85% success rate in treating cancer (AHPRA 2018).

In line with other studies (Lavorgna and Di Ronco 2018; Lavorgna and Bishop in Chapter 11 in this book), we recognise that the categorisation CAMs as benign or as potentially dangerous quackeries depends on the contextual shifting balance between the benefits (health, quality of life, psychological, spiritual) and the harms (health, emotional and psychological, financial) they can bring to people. In our study, we will focus only on those 'alternative' health approaches that are, or are likely to be, seriously harmful for the patient, with a case-by-case approach to identify them. These types of CAMs have been previously described in the literature, among other things, as '(CAM) quackeries' (Lerner 1984; Lavorgna and Di Ronco 2018), 'frauds' (Konnikova 2016; Lavorgna and Di Ronco 2017), and 'CAM-adjacent health scams' (see Chapter 11). These definitions, however, tend to suggest an element of *mens rea* (that is, the intention or knowledge of wrongdoing) that might not always be present in the provider, and hence these might not be the best terms to describe the complexity of offenders' mindsets and motivations—this is why in this study we will more broadly refer to them as harmful alternative health practices.

Indeed, previous research suggests that individuals involved in harmful alternative health practices (herein referred to as 'providers') are not part of a homogeneous group, but rather they can be very diverse, moved by very different types of motivations: some seem to search profit, social prestige, or a combination of both; others seem to be under a self-delusion of having found the 'real' treatment and wisdom (Lavorgna and Di Ronco 2017, 2018). To the authors' knowledge, so far, no systematic analysis has been carried out to develop a criminological typology of providers. Nonetheless, other sources can give us an insight into the motivations of alternative medicine providers. For instance, in the fictional but semi-autobiographical book *Confessions of a Quack*, MD Bratman (2008) describes the adventures of Holistic Harry, an MD practising alternative medicine 'on faith' who comes to realise the non-scientific value of his alternative medicine beliefs (because the treatments he proposes are based on tradition, anecdote, and authority, but they do not pass double-blind studies). This type of reading suggests that wishful thinking and idealism might be at the basis of honest mistakes done by some providers. This can be a valid explanation for the overselling of some CAMs (which would not meet any definition of fraud, as the *mens rea* requirement would be missing). However, it is self-evident that this explanation would be extremely simplistic to cover many, if not most, of the harmful alternative health practices preying on vulnerable or unwary individuals.

As anticipated above, others have attempted to frame some offenders as health fraudsters moved by profit. Konnikova (2016), for instance, in discussing the case of Belle Gibson (a former Australian wellness blogger who misled people from all over the world with her claims on how to treat cancer 'naturally', see also Lavorgna and Sugiura 2018), emphasises that she should be considered a con artist, motivated by personal gain. Konnikova reminds us that con artists often have some or all of the so-called dark triad of personality traits—psychopathy, Machiavellianism, and narcissism, thus suggesting that we might better understand health fraudsters (and maybe classify them) by looking at their personality traits.

Existing literature (mostly grounded in criminal psychology) on offender typologies can provide a solid ground to further explore and problematise the complexity of behaviours, mindsets, and characteristics of providers. This literature will be briefly presented in the following section, with a specific focus on serial killer classifications. Indeed, whilst we do not want to suggest a resemblance between serial killers and providers, we think that we can learn from the literature on serial killers as it deals with similarly complex cases, where heterogeneous types of offenders are moved by many and various motivations.

Typologies of criminal behaviour: the case of serial killers

The development of offender typologies has a long history. Cesare Lombroso is credited with developing the first general typology of offending in 1876, where he identified six types of offenders. Whilst very primitive and the focus of intense criticism, Lombroso's typology of offenders set off a wave of academic focus on the development of offender typologies in order to understand, prevent, and treat offending behaviour (Wolfgang 2006; Byrne and Roberts 2007). Indeed, etiological and diagnostic typologies can be used to identify and rehabilitate offenders, whilst typologies developed from analysing patterns in offenders and crimes can aid criminal investigations (Gibbons 1975; Kapardis and Krambia-Kapardis 2004). Since the work of Lombroso, many typologies of offenders have been developed, ranging from sexual offending (Fox and Farrington 2018) and arson (Kocsis et al. 1998; Santtila et al. 2003) to cybercrime (Warikoo 2014) and fraud (Kapardis and Krambia-Kapardis 2004; Chan et al. 2014).

Developing an offender typology of a serial killer is the most common application of typologies of criminal behaviour: there are a number of serial killer typologies that have been developed and many that attribute offending to a killer's pathology. Miller (2014) reviewed the assorted typologies of serial killers elaborated by other researchers, including those proposed by Deitz (1986, 1987), Holmes (Holmes and De Burger 1985, 1988; Holmes and Holmes 1996), and Sewall and colleagues (2013). According to Miller, there are considerable commonalities across the different typologies which indicates a level of construct validity. From these commonalities, Miller proposed an integrative classification of common serial killer subtypes: (1) sexual sadists, (2) delusional killers, (3) custodial killers, and (4) utilitarian killers.

Sexual sadists

Sexual sadists kill because they enjoy killing and get thrill and sexual gratification from torturing their victims in the process (Dietz 1986,1987; Rappaport 1988; Holmes and Holmes 1996; Myers et al. 2006; James and Proulx 2016). It has been argued that, among other things, serial sexual murderers are socially isolated, humiliated, rejected, have sexual fantasies that involve harming others or oneself, and lack healthy emotional and sexual relationships. Their modus operandi is well planned as to ensure that the murder matches their fantasies: their crimes are sadistic and organised. There is evidence to suggest that paraphilias begin at a young age; a history of animal cruelty is a common characteristic of the sexually sadistic killer, which also often begins at a young age (Johnson and Becker 1997). According to Meloy (2000), the serial sexual killer is usually male, having killed his first victim before turning 30 years old, whilst victims are typically female, unknown to the killer, and are the same ethnicity as the killer. There are many documented examples of the serial sexual sadistic killer (Jack the Ripper being probably the most famous one).

Delusional killers

According to Miller (2014), delusional killers are killers who are on some sort of mission. This can be either because they are psychotic or because they are motivated by ideology, murdering people they see as undesirable or detrimental to the human race. Holmes and colleagues (Holmes and De Burger 1985, 1988; Holmes and Holmes 1996) identified two categories that could fit into this classification of the delusional killer: the visionary serial killer, who is typically delusional and suffering from hallucinations (which are commanding him/her to kill); and the mission serial killer, who is driven by religious or political ideology and wants to cleanse the world of a particular group of people. For Holmes, this type of killer might be diagnosed as delusional or they might not have any diagnosable mental disorder. The Anders Behring Breivik case is one example where the killer strenuously denied any mental illness, believing a diagnosis would delegitimise the political message he was trying to deliver (*The Telegraph* 2012).

Utilitarian killers

Utilitarian killers are centrally concerned with financial or material gain, but can additionally be driven by anger or revenge. In the Dietz typology (1986, 1987), there are two categories which fit with the utilitarian classification: crime spree killers (for instance, Bonnie and Clyde), where robbery is often involved in the murders; and organised crime functionaries, which describes the typical hitman or political assassin, where the killers are being paid to murder a specific person. In the Holmes' typology (Holmes and De Burger 1985, 1988; Holmes and Holmes 1996), the utilitarian killer falls in the category of the comfort-oriented serial killer and includes hitmen and people who murder family members, for example, for financial gain. It is not unusual for feelings of hatred to also be fuelling the drive to murder family members. Miller (2014) discusses findings to suggest that, whilst men mostly commit serial homicides, 15% of serial murderers are female, with females being more likely to fit into this utilitarian typology or the custodial killer typology discussed next. Of course, this does not mean that utilitarian killers are more likely to be female, only that on the rare occurrence of a female serial murderer, they will likely fall into one of these two typologies, rather than the sexually sadistic killer or the delusional killer.

Custodial killers

Custodial killers generally work in a healthcare, caretaker, or parental role; their motives might include ideology, revenge, 'twisted altruism' (where they believe they are helping their victim or wider society), financial gain, or power (where they enjoy having the power to choose whether someone lives or dies) (Miller 2014:6). Some put their victims' lives in danger so they can get credit from colleagues for going to great lengths to save the person, or the crisis situation is induced in order to attract medical attention—a version of Munchausen syndrome by proxy (MSBP) (Yorker et al. 2006). One particular subtype of custodial killers works in the healthcare sector; they are also referred to as 'angels of death' or 'healthcare serial killers' (HSKs) (Yardley and Wilson 2016). It has been reported that the incidence of healthcare workers murdering, or attempting to murder, their patients has increased since the 1970s (Field and Pearson 2010; Yardley and Wilson 2016), with notable examples from the United Kingdom including Harold Shipman and Beverley Allitt.

Lubaszka and colleagues (2014) identified patterns and activities that suggest HSKs engage in a similar type of confidence game as con artists: both HSKs and con artists target and groom their victims because of their vulnerabilities, and then take advantage of them; they use manipulation and self-presentation to gain trust and to appear helpful. Whereas the con artist exchanges trust for money or other gain, HSKs exchange trust for hope; they both carefully plan their activities before, during, and after the event to avoid the likelihood of being detected (this can involve choosing methods that are less likely to draw attention). The effectiveness of the techniques adopted by HSKs is evident in the number of examples where offenders were able to operate for many years before being caught and from the fact that it was typically co-workers rather than the victim's families that raised concern: for instance, Beverly Allitt had tried to kill twins, but one lived and was left brain damaged. The parents of the children were so impressed with Allitt's efforts to save their daughter that they made Allitt godmother of their child (Lubaszka et al. 2014).

In terms of demographics, Miller argues that females are more likely to belong to the custodial or utilitarian types of killing, compared to any other category. There is also a tendency for HSKs to be portrayed as female in media representations. However, there are some relatively recent findings to challenge this gendered representation of 'angels of death'. For instance, Field and Pearson (2010) found that demographic characteristics such as gender and age revealed no typical offender. Instead, characteristics related to the killers' past experience, notably their experiences of emotional and physical abuse in childhood (which is also common in other types of serial killers) were better predictors (Field and Pearson 2010). Lubaszka et al. (2014) further report that in their analysis of cases, males were able to continue offending over longer periods, amassing more victims. Yorker et al. (2006) also report that males and females each made up half of the offending sample in their analysis. Further, they demonstrate that most HSKs are Caucasian and from the US, Germany, and England and Wales, and most are nurses rather than doctors.

These offender subtypes demonstrate the heterogeneous nature of offending. The next section of the chapter outlines the methodology used to develop our own typology of harmful non-science-based health providers. This typology—and how it relates to the offender subtypes described previously—will be outlined in the Discussion section.

Methodology

In order to access extensive information on a broad number of providers of harmful alternative health practices, we gathered data in and on the United Kingdom from a number of publicly available sources, namely newspapers articles, grey literature, and judicial material. The documents were coded manually, with relevant passages in the text categorised according to codes and sub-codes as summarised in Table 2.1. The use of documentary sources is consistent with other studies on offender typologies (Yorker et al. 2006; Field and Pearson 2010; Grugan 2018).

Newspaper articles

This study focuses on newspaper articles published in the United Kingdom over 10 years (1 January 2008–31 December 2017). Articles were extracted from *Google News*. Trying to keep the search as comprehensive as possible, the following syntaxes were chosen for the keyword searches: '* [(quack*) OR scam OR fraud] AND alternative'; '* [(quack*) OR scam OR fraud] AND medicine'; '* [(quack*) OR scam OR fraud] AND health'; '* [(quack*) OR scam OR fraud] AND natural'. The search was entered based on the following criteria: timeframe (01/01/2008–31/12/2017); country (UK); type (all news); sort by relevance. After these preliminary keyword searches, articles were manually sorted to exclude those non-relevant for the scope of this study (e.g., articles focusing on counterfeited pharmaceuticals; articles on generic 'slimming pills' without any reference to potentially harmful alternative health practices; articles dismissive of CAMs in general, or without reference to a specific case/provider) and to eliminate duplicates. A total of 57 press items were identified as relevant for the analysis.

Grey literature

We searched for additional case studies in websites and, when available, in reports published by a variety of potentially relevant institutions, and specifically the Medicines and Healthcare products Regulatory Agency; Citizens Advice; the Scams Team at the National Trading Standards; Action Fraud; the Royal Pharmaceutical Society; the Information Commissioner's Office (no relevant results were found in any of these); the Adverting Standard Authority (where we found 18 relevant cases within its rulings 01/01/2008–31/12/2017); relevant charities and debunking websites, namely Think Jessica, DC's Improbable Science, The Nightingale Collaboration, The Quackometer, and Sense About Science (where we found a total of 33 relevant cases). We also checked the websites of legit CAMs associations[2] and of the Complementary and Natural Healthcare Council,[3] but we could not find anything relevant, with the exception of two cases respectively in the websites of the General Chiropractic Council and the General Osteopathic Council.

Judicial material

Judicial material (mostly judgements, full transcripts whenever possible) was obtained after preliminary searches on three major databases (*The Law Pages*, *Westlaw*, and *LexisNexis*) and requests to the relevant courts. We maintained the same timeframe (01/01/2008–31/12/2017), but the keyword searches were slightly different to adapt them to the different characteristics of the databases. In total, we collected judicial material for four relevant cases. Initial searches by legal categories on *The Law Pages* (fraud/attempted fraud; trade and licensing offence; misleading advertising/marketing; offences relating to fake goods; medicine/fraud; health, scam; fraudulent, health) did not lead to relevant results. Therefore, we carried out searches based on the names of key actors we identified via the media sources, which led us to the identification of one of the sampled cases. On *Westlaw*, we used the following keyword searches ('quack', 200 results; 'fraud AND health AND alternative AND medicine', 875 results; 'integrative AND medicine', 5 results; 'complementary AND medicine', 77 results) and searches by themes ('complementary and alternative medicine', 52 results; 'consent to treatment', 281 results). We manually scrutinised the results and identified four relevant cases within our timeframe. Finally, we carried out keyword searches on *LexisNexis* ('[quack OR fraud OR scam] AND health', 993 results; 'alternative medicine', 44 results), which led us to identify one new case and to collect additional material for one case identified before. We contacted the courts involved to gain access to further transcripts and were successful for one of our selected cases.

Table 2.1 Coding framework

Codes	*Sub-codes (number of references identified after eliminating duplicates)*
Provider	Named person (52) Named company (25) Named association/network of therapists/clinic/charity/homeopathic pharmacy/educational institutions (15) Non-identified (but the document analysed refers to a specific individual, e.g., 'a therapist', 'a healer', 'an osteomyologist', etc. (11))
Demographic characteristics of the provider	Age (specified only in 11 cases, in years: 35; 39; 39; 45; 52; 53; 54; 56; 60; 62; 77) Gender (M = 34; F = 20)
	Occupation/qualification (yoga teacher: 1; pharmacist: 1; qualified nurse: 1; discredited former doctors: 2; scientific graduates: 3; 'healers': 4; GPs: 4; fake doctors: 5; nutritionists: 7; doctors running a private practice: 8; CAM practitioners, or presenting themselves as such: 20)
	Nationality (specified only in 6 cases: British; Irish; Slovakian; Mexican; Australian; German-American. From the context it can be supposed that the overwhelming majority of the other providers are British national and/or resident)

Codes	*Sub-codes (number of references identified after eliminating duplicates)*
Organisation	One person (43)
	Couple (3)
	Group (if 3 or more) (n/a)
Motivation	Financial profit (48)
	Desire to be credited (17)
	Genuine belief to help people (10)
	Holistic belief (5)
	Sexual motivation (3)
	Conspiratorial belief (2)
	Negligence/recklessness (1)
	Possible mental disorder after a trauma (1)
	Antagonistic attitude against science-based medicine (6)

Results

Providers, their demographic characteristics, and their organisation

Through our sources we identified 52 distinct named providers, plus smaller numbers of non-identifiable providers, named companies, associations, clinics, pharmacies, and other institutions directly selling or otherwise offering (potentially) harmful health practices—for a total of 103 relevant actors. It is important to underline that most of the information presented in the following analysis does not focus on the named companies, as from the sources it was not possible to have enough understanding of the characteristics and organisational features of those running the company (e.g., a company might be managed by a single individual).

As regards the demographic characteristics, the data (although very limited) suggest a prevalence of middle-aged adults, followed by young adults. As providers might be active for years, it is likely that deviant behaviour starts in early adulthood. There is a prevalence of male offenders, who come from a wide range of professions from both the modern scientific and CAM-related health sectors; we identified as male all the 'healers' and the fake and discredited doctors encountered in the analysis, which suggests a prevalence of men in the more 'extreme' cases. With a single exception (the wife in a criminal couple, who according to judicial data acted under the 'malevolent influence' of her husband), all the women identified were GPs, nurses, or CAM practitioners practising traditional/recognised forms of alternative treatments (e.g., acupuncturist, herbalist, naturopath) or other health-related practices (e.g., nutritionist). However, they were bringing it too far, for instance by advocating a specific diet to treat diseases or conditions such as autism (often while questioning vaccine safety). In two cases the female providers are described as mums of autistic children, and in one case a male provider is described as the dad of one of his patients. Most providers come from/are based in the local communities in which they operate and seem to be well-integrated in those communities.

It is interesting to note that a majority of providers are CAM practitioners, followed by doctors (most of them running a private practice, but some operating in the National Health Service). The category 'CAM practitioners', however, covers also those self-presenting themselves as such, but who might be considered outliers by their colleagues—something to keep in mind when debating the necessity to regulate CAMs and the professionalisation of CAM practitioners (Clarke et al. 2004; Kelner et al. 2004; Ijaz and Boon 2018). Nutritionists (a title that in many countries, including the United Kingdom, is not subject to professional regulation) follows. There are then cases of fake doctors, 'healers' (sometimes self-named 'bishops' or other labels evoking a religious/spiritual element), graduates in scientific disciplines, discredited former doctors (who continue to operate as providers of harmful alternative health practices despite being struck off the British medical register), a qualified nurse, a pharmacist, and a yoga teacher.

The majority of providers seem to be operating alone (in a few cases the provider was presented as operating in a clinic or pharmacy, but this does not prove the presence of a structured organisational form as he/she might be the only provider in said clinic). When operating in a group, providers still seem to enjoy a certain autonomy: a few associations and networks of therapists were reported in the news, but also in this case we cannot conclusively say that a structured organisation is in place, as these networks and associations might be used by one or two providers to give themselves an aura of legitimacy and sophistication. From the analysis emerges a certain amount of professionalism in the activities carried out: they often entail preparatory activities and are generally carried out over a prolonged period, often years or even decades. Among the preparatory activities, we could distinguish different forms of advertisement, the set-up of clinics and companies, and the organisation of conferences where therapeutic approaches are promoted and self-published books are presented.

Interestingly, we found 20 additional references (in the analysis of newspaper articles) of media and sport celebrities, as well as politicians, praising potentially harmful alternative health practices. Not to exceed the scope of this chapter, we will not focus on the role of famous testimonials in promoting medical misinformation; nonetheless, it is worth noting that their media presence is in line with what was found in recent analyses of media representations of alternative medicine (Lavorgna and Di Ronco 2018; Lavorgna and Bishop in Chapter 11), and their responsibility in drawing vulnerable readers closer to harmful practices and practitioners certainly deserves further attention and research.

Motivations

Financial profit is explicitly reported as the main motivation for providers in an overwhelming majority of news (e.g., '[he] lives a life of luxury founded on a model of encouraging desperate families to raise hundreds of thousands of pounds . . . and then gives them worthless treatments that often extend suffering'). This is in line with the prevalence of the economic frame in British media in reporting CAM-related health scams, where perpetrators are depicted as con artists cashing in on the desperation of vulnerable patients (see Chapter 11).

Another prevalent motivation is the desire to be credited—that is, to receive validation and legitimation not only for the work done, but also and foremost for the identity they have built. Thus, training centres in alternative medicine which do not confer any legal qualification are named 'faculties' and 'colleges' ('She claimed that her PhD came from the American College of Nutrition, but it turned out to come from a correspondence course from a non-accredited US "college"'); in providers' clinics and houses we find 'certificates boasting [their] many qualifications' (such as diplomas in disciplines such as 'holistic nutritional practice' or 'naturopathic iridology'). Some providers present themselves as doctors even when they are not ('With . . . the title "Dr" you might be forgiven for thinking that [she] is a medically trained doctor. She is not. But she describes herself as a "practitioner of health in its broadest sense", although not so broad as to be an actual qualified medical doctor'). Some dress up for the role, in a way that is probably meant to reassure potential patients ('Dressed in his white medical smock, with half-rimmed glasses perched on the end of his nose, Dr . . . appears the stereotypical wise and helpful practitioner').

Interestingly, the specificities of some cases suggest that some providers do genuinely believe that they are helping their patients, as in the case of a mother (and doctor) using the same contested health approach for her children (e.g., 'She's a parent of a child with autism, so it would be hard to believe her motivations are anything but genuine'). A homeopathic pharmacist was reportedly dispensing homeopathic whooping cough vaccines also to his own children. In another case for which we could access judicial material, a CAM practitioner offering treatments of reiki, aromatherapy, and reflexology became the victim of his own practice. After discovering he had diabetes and an infected wound led him to gangrene and septicaemia, he decided not to accept conventional medical help, which led to his death.

In a minority of cases we found the presence of a sexual motivation to the crime. For one of these cases we could access some of the judicial files and therefore had more in-depth information. The main offender was running an alternative therapy clinic at his home, with the help of his wife. He deliberately misdiagnosed the women approaching him for help with medical problems as suffering from cancer. Then, under the pretence of administering beneficial treatment, he subjected his victims to penetrative sexual assault.

Some providers are motivated by strong inner beliefs and opinions, and specifically by holistic beliefs (e.g., 'as a spiritual healer, I believe that cancer is connected to the soul and to the life content of a sufferer') or by conspiratorial beliefs, with the consequence that they end up not trusting and believing the 'official' healthcare system (e.g., '[he] also runs an organisation . . . which predicts the destruction of the world in a Third World War and says that 9/11 was a US government plot'). Indeed, some providers display an antagonistic attitude against science-based medicine (e.g., 'Most doctors don't listen to patients and don't want to consider views that undermine their authority'; 'I have faced

11 years of GMC [General Medical Council] prosecution simply because my ideas on medicine lie outside conventional medical practice. At least I have to be thankful that I live in the 21st century—earlier heretics were burnt at the stake!'; 'Probably the worst person to ask about this is your oncologist').

Finally, we identified isolated cases where it is suggested that behind the actions of a provider there is a possible mental disorder after a traumatic event (e.g., 'he approaches the dead body, sees the dead soul and realises he has some magic powers of some sort'), or negligence/recklessness (e.g., 'I know it should not say anything that says we are treating cancer ... I don't know how [a video strap line that included the word "cured" for a tumour treatment] got there.... I don't write on my website, I have other people update it for me. I was checking the website, but obviously not everything that went on there').

Discussion

From the results of our analysis, we could identify some parallelisms among the many and various motivations at the heart of the activities of providers, and Miller's classification. On this basis, we propose a provider typology based on the following four subtypes: (1) utilitarian providers; (2) custodial providers (with the subtypes 'good-faith' providers and 'the egotistical fake' providers); (3) sexual abusers; and (4) delusional providers.

Utilitarian providers are moved mainly by the desire to obtain financial profit, and they can amass significant material gain from fraudulent practices. An element of fraud, indeed, is generally present, as these providers are aware that the treatment they propose are worthless. Simply, they do not care about the consequences of their actions. There are clear parallels with the utilitarian killer who kills for material gain; of course, for utilitarian providers the material gain would not typically be achieved by a killing per se (the death of the patient might not even occur) but by the fraudulent methods employed that leads to the payment of disproportionate amount of money for useless or potentially dangerous treatments.

Custodial providers have a recognised authoritative role and are in a position of power in comparison to their patients—who trust them, literally, with their lives. Generally, custodial providers do not want to cause harm, but harm is a by-product of their actions. Depending on their predominant motivation, we can distinguish two distinct subtypes within this group. First, *'good-faith' providers* are those who genuinely believe that they are helping the victim. They are generally health practitioners, working in modern scientific or CAM-related health sectors. The element of 'good-faith', of course, does not mean that they do not bear responsibility for their acts (even in those cases where their responsibility 'only' lies in overselling the therapeutic value of an alternative treatment)—responsibility that could be addressed as negligence or abuse of trust (that bond of trust at the basis of their relationship with their patients) at the minimum. We can identify here a limited parallelism with custodial killers, and more precisely with those 'angels of death' moved by mercy, who might genuinely believe that they are helping the victim by ending their suffering (even if this belief may be delusional).

Second, *'the egotistical fake' providers* strive for receiving credit, validation, and legitimation: they have built/are building an identity around their work as providers, often peddling degrees and accreditations or presenting themselves as certified health practitioners while they are not. Nonetheless, their position towards their victims remains one of power, as their victims trust them and recognise them as health authorities. Here, a limited parallelism can be drawn with those custodial killers motivated by power and a desire for their life-saving efforts to be praised as heroic by their colleagues and by the family of their victims.

Sexual abusers have a sexual motivation to the crime; a major reason for them to act as providers is to have access to vulnerable victims, and the treatment offered being a means to the sexual assault. It is possible that providers will show similarities with the sadistic killer; for instance, if they take pleasure in conning and harming the people that turn to them for help.

Finally, *delusional providers* believe themselves to be on a mission to heal or to rid the world/their social circles of westernised, science-based medicine, and/or 'big-pharma' influences. As in the case of the delusional killer, they might be moved by an ideological desire to protect the world from undesirable people (e.g., providers holding conspiratorial beliefs), or they might be psychotic.

Concluding remarks

This chapter has developed a typology of providers of harmful non-science-based health practices. The typology presented here has four categories: utilitarian providers, custodial providers, sexual providers, and delusional providers. Each category of provider demonstrates different motivations for committing harmful non-science-based health practices; motivations that have been linked to the classification of common serial killer subtypes. In addition to these typologies, a tentative discussion of the demographics and organisation of providers has been presented. The analysis demonstrated that there is a prevalence of middle-aged, male providers, whilst many providers are CAM practitioners and doctors. The results also indicate that providers are well-organised, professional, and integrated into their communities.

This chapter should be regarded as a starting point for the further development of a criminological typology of harmful non-science-based health providers, which we hope could serve as a framework to filter the different experiences of similar dangerous practices in other countries, thus facilitating comparative research. Additional research—more in-depth analyses based on different types of data, such as interviews with providers—is required in order to better understand the motivations and aetiology of providers. Further, the issue of the relationship between providers and their communities could be a point of exploration for future research. For instance, if we continue to draw parallels to serial killer typologies, the FBI typology of organised versus disorganised offender typology suggests that organised offenders would usually offend further away from home to reduce their chances of being caught (Ressler et al. 1986, 1988). However, the providers in the current analysis were organised yet operating from their own communities. Thus, it would be useful for further research to explore the reasons for this; for instance, is it because they believe in what they are doing, because it helps them seem more trustworthy to their victims, or for purely logistic reasons? Also, are there particular types of communities or social organisation that are susceptible to the influence of harmful non-science-based health providers? Such questions are important if we are to develop a useful typology to aid our understanding of the harms caused by providers, the motivations behind their actions, and to develop prevention strategies to minimise harm.

Acknowledgements

We would like to thank the late Laura Little for her precious contribution in the data collection of judicial data, and Eleanor Lambourn for her valuable help in collecting data from the media. This study has been supported by the Strategic Interdisciplinary Research Development Fund, Faculty of Social Sciences, University of Southampton.

Notes

1 We use the term 'criminological types' here instead of the term 'offender typology' because some of the providers of harmful non-science-based health practices discussed in this chapter will not have been identified as an offender by the criminal justice system.
2 As listed in www.citizensadvice.org.uk/health/private-healthcare/private-healthcare1/alternative-medicine-organisations/.
3 That is, the British register for complementary healthcare practitioners who have met certain standards, which was set up in 2008 with government funding and support to protect the public.

References

AHPRA (2018) AHPRA successfully prosecutes fake Queensland chiropractor. Available at: www.chiropracticboard.gov.au/news/2018-02-06-ahpra-successfully-prosecutes-fake-qld-chir.aspx

Angell M and Kassirer JP (1998) Alternative medicine: the risks of untested and unregulated remedies. *New England Journal of Medicine* 339(12):839–841

Bashford EF (1911) Cancer, credulity and quackery. *The British Medical Journal* 1(2630):1221–1230

Bratman S (2008) *Confessions of a quack.* Available at: www.mendosa.com/Confessions.pdf

Byrne JM and Roberts AR (2007) New directions in offender typology design, development, and implementation: can we balance risk, treatment and control? *Aggression and Violent Behavior* 12(5):483–492

Chan V, Chow KP, Kwan M, Fong G, Hui M and Tang J (2014) An exploratory profiling study of online auction fraudsters. In Peterson G and Shenoi S (eds.) *Advances in digital forensics X: IFIP advances in information and communication technology*, vol. 433. Berlin: Springer

Clarke DB, Marcus AD and Segrott J (2004) No alternative? The regulation and professionalisation of complementary and alternative medicine in the United Kingdom. *Health & Place* 10(4):329–338

Delgado-López P and Corrales-García E (2018) Influence of internet and social media in the promotion of alternative oncology, cancer quackery, and the predatory publishing phenomenon. *Cureus* 10(5):e2617

Dietz PE (1986) Mass, serial and sensational homicides: the investigative perspective. *Bulletin of the New York Academy of Medicine* 62(5):492–496

Dietz PE (1987) Patterns in human violence. *Psychiatric Update: American Psychiatric Association Annual Review* 6:465–490

EFCAM (2017) *CAM definition*. European Federation for Complementary and Alternative Medicine. Available at: http://www.efcam.eu/cam/cam-definition/Ernst E (2011) Integrative medicine: smuggling alternative practices into rational medicine? *Focus on Alternative and Complementary Therapies* 16(1):1–2

Ernst E, Pittler MH and Wider B (2001) *The desktop guide to complementary and alternative medicine*. London: Mosby

Field J and Pearson A (2010) Caring to death: the murder of patients by nurses. *International Journal of Nursing Practice* 16(3):301–309

Fox B and Farrington DP (2018) What have we learned from offender profiling? A systematic review and meta-analysis of 40 years of research. *Psychological Bulletin* 144(12):1247–127

Gibbons DC (1975) Offender typologies – two decades later. *British Journal of Criminology* 15(2):140–156

Grugan ST (2018) The companions we keep: a situational analysis and proposed typology of companion animal cruelty offenses. *Deviant Behavior* 39(9):1153–1169

Holmes MM, Bishop FL and Calman L (2017) 'I just googled and read everything': exploring breast cancer survivors' use of the internet to find information on complementary medicine. *Complementary Therapies in Medicine* 33:78–84

Holmes RM and De Burger J (1985) Profiles in terror: the serial murderer. *Federal Probation* 39:29–34

Holmes RM and De Burger J (1988) *Serial murder*. Newbury Park: Sage

Holmes RM and Holmes ST (1996) *Profiling violent crimes: an investigative tool*. Thousand Oaks: Sage

Ijaz N and Boon H (2018) Statutory regulation of traditional medicine practitioners and practices: the need for distinct policy making guidelines. *The Journal of Alternative and Complementary Medicine* 24(4)

James J and Proulx J (2016) The modus operandi of serial and nonserial sexual murderers: a systematic review. *Aggression and Violent Behavior* 31:200–218

Johnson BR and Becker JV (1997) Natural born killers? The development of the sexually sadistic serial killer. *The Journal of the American Academy of Psychiatry and the Law* 25(3):335–348

Kapardis A and Krambia-Kapardis M (2004) Enhancing fraud prevention and detection by profiling fraud offenders. *Criminal Behaviour and Mental Health* 14(3):189–201

Kelner M, Wellman B, Boon H and Welsh S (2004) Responses of established healthcare to the professionalization of complementary and alternative medicine in Ontario. *Social Sciences & Medicine* 59(5):915–930

Kocsis RN, Irwin HJ and Hayes AF (1998) Organised and disorganised criminal behaviour syndromes in arsonists: a validation study of a psychological profiling concept. *Psychiatry, Psychology and Law* 5(1):117–131

Konnikova M (2016) Mind games: how con artists get the better of you. *New Scientist*. Jan 20

Lavorgna A and Bishop FL (2017) Exploring health scams in the UK: an interdisciplinary perspective. Final workshop, project 'Hush the quacks. Exploring health fraud scams in the UK', University of Southampton. Sep 5, 2017

Lavorgna A and Di Ronco A (2017) Fraud victims or unwary accomplices? An exploratory study of online communities supporting quack medicine. In van Duyne PC, Harvey J, Antonopoulos GA and von Lampe K (eds.) *The many faces of crime for profit and ways of tackling it*. Oisterwijk, NL: Wolf Legal Publishers

Lavorgna A and Di Ronco A (2018) Media representations of complementary and alternative medicine in the Italian press: a criminological perspective. *European Journal of Criminology* 15(4):421–441

Lavorgna A and Sugiura L (2018) Caught in a lie: the rise and fall of a respectable deviant. *Deviant Behavior* (online first)

Lerner IJ (1984) The whys of cancer quackery. *Cancer* 53:815–819

Lubaszka CK, Shon PC and Hinch R (2014) Healthcare serial killers as confidence men. *Journal of Investigative Psychology and Offender Profiling* 11(1):1–28

Meloy JR (2000) The nature and dynamics of sexual homicide: an integrative review. *Aggression and Violent Behavior* 5(1):1–22

Miller L (2014) Serial killers: I. Subtypes, patterns, and motives. *Aggression and Violent Behavior* 19(1):1–11

Myers WC, Husted DS, Safarik ME and O'Toole ME (2006) The motivation behind serial sexual homicide: is it sex, power, and control, or anger? *Journal of Forensic Sciences* 51(4):900–907

Offit P (2013) *Killing us softly: the sense and nonsense of alternative medicine*. London: Harper Collins

Rappaport RG (1988) The serial and mass murderer. *American Journal of Forensic Psychiatry* 9:39–48

Ressler RK, Burgess AW and Douglas JE (1988) *Sexual homicide: patterns and motives*. New York: Free Press

Ressler RK, Burgess AW, Douglas JE, Hartman CR and D'Agostino RB (1986) Serial killers and their victims: identifying patterns through crime scene analysis. *International Journal of Violence* 1:288–308

Santtila P, Häkkänen H and Fritzon K (2003) Inferring the characteristics of an arsonist from crime scene actions: a case study in offender profiling. *International Journal of Police Science & Management* 5(1):1–15

Sewall LA, Krupp DB and Lalumiere ML (2013) A test of two typologies of sexual homicide. *Sex Abuse* 25(1):82–100

The Telegraph (2012) Norway killer Anders Behring Breivik claims there is a 'racist plot' to discredit him as insane. Available at: www.telegraph.co.uk/news/worldnews/europe/norway/9221345/Norway-killer-Anders-Behring-Breivik-claims-there-is-a-racist-plot-to-discredit-him-as-insane.html

Warikoo A (2014) Proposed methodology for cybercriminal profiling. *Information Security Journal* 23(4–6):172–178

Wells RE, Bertisch SM, Buettner C, Phillips RS and McCarthy EP (2011) Complementary and alternative medicine use among adults with migraines/severe headaches. *Headache* 51(7):1087–1097

Wolfgang ME (2006) Pioneers in criminology: Cesare Lombroso (1835–1909). *The Journal of Criminal Law, Criminology, and Police Science* 52(4):361

Yardley E and Wilson D (2016) In search of the 'angels of death': conceptualising the contemporary nurse healthcare serial killer. *Journal of Investigative Psychology and Offender Profiling* 13(1):39–55

Yorker BC, Kizer KW, Lampe P, Forrest AR, Lannan JM and Russell DA (2006) Serial murder by healthcare professionals. *Journal of Forensic Sciences* 51(6):1362–1371

Zhang Y, Dennis J, Leach M, Bishop FL, Cramer H, Chung V, Moore C, Lauche R, Cook R, Sibbritt D and Adams J (2017) Complementary and alternative medicine use among US Adults with headache or migraine: results from the 2012 national health interview survey. *Headache* 57(8):1228–1242

3 Science denial

Psychological processes underlying denial of science-based medical practices

Sara Prot and Craig A. Anderson

Introduction

> *Unvaccinated children are much healthier than vaccinated children. You can line up the doctors from here to down the block refuting me, but I'm not gonna change my mind.*
>
> Sarah Pope, blogger, *The Daily Show* interview, 2014

Overwhelming scientific evidence supports the safety of vaccinations (Maglione et al. 2014), dangers of tobacco use (Landman and Glantz 2009), and science-based prevention and treatment strategies for HIV/AIDS (Bogart et al. 2008). Nonetheless, public opinion frequently is incongruent with the scientific consensus. Individuals and groups continue to doubt and deny scientific findings in various areas. Denial of science, sometimes also labeled 'denialism' or 'rejection of science', can be defined as dismissal of established scientific evidence for non-scientific reasons (Lewandowsky et al. 2013d; Diethelm and McKee 2009). It is important to distinguish denial from scientific skepticism. Genuine scientific skepticism is based on relevant theoretical predictions and empirical evidence. It is an integral part of the scientific method and leads to reliable and valid conclusions (Jacques 2012). On the other hand, science denial is often unaffected by accurate scientific information, persevering even in the face of overwhelming empirical evidence and clear scientific consensus (Lewandowsky et al. 2013d).

In some cases, denialist beliefs are innocuous. For example, some of the members of the Flat Earth Society (which currently consists of over 500 people from the US, the UK, and other countries) still sincerely believe that the earth is a flat disc surrounded by a 150-foot wall of ice at its outer edge (The Flat Earth Society 2019). In other cases, science denial costs lives. Despite clear scientific evidence supporting the effectiveness and safety of vaccinations (Maglione et al. 2014), unfounded concerns about potential harmful side effects of vaccines led a number of parents in the US and the UK to delay or refuse vaccination (Poland and Spier 2010). Clusters of intentionally under-vaccinated children have triggered outbreaks of vaccine-preventable diseases such as pertussis (Atwell et al. 2013) and measles (Sugerman et al. 2010), causing a major public health risk. A tragic example of what can happen when science denial is governmentally supported can be observed in post-apartheid South Africa. President Mbeki championed a small group of AIDS denialists who claimed that AIDS is caused by poverty and malnutrition, not by HIV (Bateman 2007). Mbeki's government recommended local vegetables as a treatment for AIDS and banned the use of antiretroviral drugs in public hospitals, promoting the idea that antivirals are a part of a white conspiracy to reduce the black African population. These inappropriate policies guided by science denial are thought to be responsible for around 171,000 HIV infections and 343,000 deaths between 1999 and 2007. Examples such as these leave no doubt that science denial is dangerous—it can endanger lives of both denialists and non-denialists.

An intriguing aspect of science denial is that it is often accompanied by anger and aggression towards scientists. Researchers from a wide range of disciplines have reported being targeted by similar kinds of personal and professional attacks, including complaints, legal threats, intimidation, cyber-bullying, and public abuse (Lewandowsky et al. 2013c). Some of these aggressive strategies are highly organized—e.g., the tactics used by the tobacco industry to discredit researchers and cast doubt on the evidence that smoking causes cancer (Landman and Glantz 2009; Nature 2010). Other aggressive actions (such as insulting email messages) seem more impulsive, have the immediate goal to hurt scientists personally, and seem to be rooted in denialists' feelings of anger and hostility in response to threatening research findings (Lewandowsky et al. 2013a; Nauroth et al. 2014). Both types of attacks can have far-reaching negative consequences: personal attacks cause emotional distress and take up time, interfering with researchers' work, whereas organized professional attacks have the potential to derail the scientific process by delaying or stopping publication of manuscripts (Lewandowsky et al. 2013c).

What factors and processes lead to science denial? According to the public irrationality thesis (Kahan 2013), denial stems from a lack of comprehension of scientific methods and evidence among the general public. The deficit model of science communication assumes that increased communication about scientific issues will lead to a shift in public opinion toward scientific consensus (Hart and Nisbet 2011). However, a number of studies suggest that this is not always the case. In fact, providing scientific evidence sometimes backfires, causing denialists to become even more entrenched in their initial beliefs and behaviors (Hart and Nisbet 2011; Lord et al. 1979). For example, Nyhan and colleagues (2014) tested interventions intended to reduce vaccine misperceptions among parents and increase vaccination rates. The pro-vaccine messages did not work as planned—some of the messages actually decreased intent to vaccinate among parents who held the most negative attitudes towards vaccination.

This research demonstrates that science denial is not a simple product of deficits in information or understanding of scientific methodology. Instead, more complex psychological processes are at play. Several areas of research in psychology help explain the roots of denial and elucidate why simply bombarding denialists with accurate scientific information does not lead to attitude change (see also Chapter 12).

Table 3.1 Factors and mechanisms leading to science denial

Individual	*Group*	*Intergroup*
Belief perseverance	Threatened social identity	Intergroup emotions
Confirmation bias, myside bias	Values and ideology	Intergroup threat
Cognitive dissonance	Cultural cognition	Intergroup conflict
Reactance	System justification	
'Forbidden fruit' effects	Social dominance orientation	
Boomerang effects (aka 'backfire effects')		
Defensiveness, the psychological immune system		
Self-affirmation		
Conspiratorial thinking		
Scientific expertise, training in research methods and rational thinking		

This chapter reviews the psychological mechanisms that lead to science denial (shown in Table 3.1), including processes affecting individuals (such as belief perseverance, confirmation bias, and cognitive dissonance), groups (such as social identification), and intergroup relations (such as intergroup threat). Special attention is given to predictors of angry denial and aggressive actions towards scientists. Finally, avenues for prevention and intervention are reviewed that can help combat science denial and reduce the risk of non-science-based medical practices.

Individual-level mechanisms leading to science denial

A rich research literature in the fields of cognitive and social psychology reveals a number of individual-level factors that contribute to science denial. The review presented here is not meant to be extensive—it highlights seven individual-level processes key to understanding science denial: (1) belief perseverance; (2) confirmation bias and myside bias; (3) reactance, boomerang effects, and 'forbidden fruit effects'; (4) cognitive dissonance; (5) defensiveness, the psychological immune system, and self-affirmation; (6) conspiratorial thinking; and (7) training in research methods and rational thinking. Illustrations are given both from empirical studies and from real-life examples of science denial.

Belief perseverance

People tend to cling strongly to their prior beliefs about how the world works—their *social theories*—even when such beliefs are no longer warranted (Anderson 1983; Anderson and Kellam 1992). Initial perceptions, opinions, and attitudes persevere in the face of disconfirming evidence. For example, Anderson et al. (1980) informed participants that a positive or negative association exists between risk taking and firefighters' job performance. Some were led to believe that high risk-takers made better firefighters; others were led to believe the opposite was true. Participants continued to believe that a true relationship exists between risk preference and job performance even when they were told that the initial information was fabricated.

Paradoxically, stronger belief perseverance occurs after exposure to weak but vivid and concrete case history data rather than stronger but abstract statistical summaries (Anderson 1983). These effects are mediated, at least in part, by the accessibility of causal explanations and formulation of causal scripts (Anderson 1983; Anderson et al. 1985). After being given the initial information, people spontaneously generate causal explanations for it. Causal explanations can then become independent of the data on which they were originally based and fuel people's beliefs even once the initial evidence is refuted (Anderson et al. 1980; Anderson 1983; McFarland et al. 2007).

A tragic real-life example of belief perseverance occurred when Andrew Wakefield and colleagues (1998) published a paper suggesting that measles-mumps-rubella (MMR) vaccine causes autism. Numerous subsequent studies using larger samples and stronger methodology disproved this finding (Taylor et al. 1999; Gerber and Offit 2009). Furthermore, an award-winning investigation by *Sunday Times* reporter Brian Deer revealed evidence of fraud—Wakefield misreported findings and had failed to disclose considerable financial conflicts of interest (Deer 2004). Finally, the Wakefield article was retracted from the *Lancet* (The Editors of the Lancet 2010). Despite these developments, panicked parents in the UK, the US, and many other countries have continued to fear that vaccinations may increase the risk of autism, leading them to delay or stop vaccinating their children (Poland and Spier 2010). A single fraudulent publication led to widespread risk to public health.

Confirmation bias, myside bias

A set of phenomena closely related to belief perseverance are confirmation biases. People tend to perceive, interpret, and use information that confirms their beliefs, while ignoring disconfirming information (Klayman and Ha 1987; Kleiman and Hassin 2013). Confirmation biases help fuel belief perseverance by prompting people to find evidence that supports views, while overlooking evidence that supports a different position.

In a classic demonstration of these processes, Lord et al. (1979) showed supporters and opponents of capital punishment two supposed studies, one that proved and one that disproved their existing belief. Both proponents and opponents of capital punishment rated the results and procedures that confirmed their own beliefs to be more convincing and better conducted. Reading this mixed evidence made them more confident in their beliefs and led to polarization of their attitudes instead of convergence.

A subtype of confirmation biases especially relevant to science denial is myside bias—the tendency to evaluate evidence and test hypotheses in a way that is biased towards one's own opinions (Stanovich et al. 2013). Unfortunately, it seems that myside bias is one of the rare cognitive processes that are completely independent of intelligence (Stanovich and West 2008; Stanovich et al. 2013). For instance, smokers underestimate health risks of secondhand smoke, heavy alcohol drinkers underestimate health risks of alcohol consumption, and these biases are not attenuated by cognitive ability (Stanovich and West 2008).

Reactance

When people feel that their freedom to engage in a behavior is threatened, they experience an aversive state of arousal (reactance) and are motivated to restore that freedom (Brehm and Brehm 1981). Therefore, if scientific findings threaten people's sense of freedom, they are likely to be denied. For instance, warning labels on tobacco products have been found to be ineffective and even lead to forbidden fruit effects, making the forbidden item more attractive to consumers (Willemsen and De Zwart 1999).

Psychological reactance also leads to behavioral change. People attempt to reaffirm their freedom by acting in opposition to a perceived threat to freedom. Results by the previously mentioned study of pro-vaccination messages by Nyhan and colleagues (2014) can also be interpreted within the framework of reactance theory. It is possible that anti-vaccination parents experienced persuasive messages as a threat to their personal freedom and responded by reducing their intentions to vaccinate.

Cognitive dissonance

Classic research within the framework of cognitive dissonance theory (Festinger 1957) is highly relevant to understanding science denial. For example, a number of studies examined cognitive dissonance among smokers and found that smokers reduce the dissonance produced by the realization that they are engaging in a risky behavior by underestimating risks of smoking and questioning the validity of studies linking smoking with negative health consequences (Lawton and Goldman 1961; Feather 1962, 1963; Pervin and Yatko 1965; Johnson 1968). One might hope that, in more recent decades, increased public awareness of risks associated with smoking would have made science denial an untenable means of dissonance reduction. Unfortunately, newer studies in this area demonstrate that this is not the case—in spite of increased awareness of scientific evidence, smokers still tend to underestimate the health risks associated with smoking (Gibbons et al. 1991, 1997).

Defensiveness, the psychological immune system, and self-affirmation

People strive to maintain their perceived worth and integrity and respond defensively to information that threatens a valued self-image (Sherman and Cohen 2006). We have a 'psychological immune system' that uses various cognitive strategies and distortions, enabling us to interpret a situation as less threatening to personal worth and well-being.

Defensive processing fuels science denial, as shown by research examining responses to threatening health information (Reed and Aspinwall 1998; Harris and Napper 2005). In one set of such studies, sexually active students responded to AIDS prevention films by lowering their perceptions of risk for sexually transmitted diseases (Morris and Swann 1996). Highest threat was experienced in response to films that depicted HIV-positive individuals who were similar to the viewers. Authors concluded that AIDS prevention films might trigger denial, especially when they hit 'too close to home'.

How can such defensiveness be reduced? Promising results have been obtained by researchers working within the framework of self-affirmation theory. People are more willing to examine and accept threatening information when their self-worth is strengthened by an affirmation of another part of their identity (e.g., receiving positive feedback about a valued self-image or writing about a value important to them, see Sherman and Cohen 2006). Self-affirmation enables people to cope with threatening information and maintain their self-worth without resorting to defensive responses, increasing the effectiveness of health messages. For instance, in a study by Sherman et al. (2000), self-affirmed participants were more receptive to health messages about HIV and purchased condoms more often.

Similarly, priming secure attachment thoughts and memories can temporarily reduce negative outgroup emotions and thereby reduce harmful behaviors and interactions with outgroup people (Saleem et al. 2015). For example: having people imagine a scene with a close friend; recall a time when someone close to them was available, supportive, and loving; or visualize a person 'who accepts and loves you and helps you in times of need' decreases the tendency to use their negative social theories about outgroup members.

Conspiratorial thinking

Conspiratorial thinking, or conspiracist ideation, involves explaining events as a result of secret machinations of powerful people or organizations (Lewandowsky et al. 2013d). A number of authors have pointed to conspiracist ideation as a key predictor of science denial (Diethelm and McKee 2009; Lewandowsky et al. 2013b). Endorsement of conspiracy theories predicts opposition to a number of well-established scientific findings, including doubts about vaccine safety, disbelief in climate change, and rejection of the link between tobacco and cancer and of the link between HIV and AIDS (Lewandowsky et al. 2013a).

Several mechanisms have been proposed that may underlie the relationship between conspiracist ideation and science denial. Whereas scientists use disconfirming evidence to reject hypotheses and revise theories, such information is often viewed as confirmation of a conspiracy theory by its followers (Lewandowsky et al. 2013b). The peer-review process is interpreted as a system of censorship (Diethelm and McKee 2009). Because of this, researchers recommend battling conspiracist ideation via indirect means, such as using self-affirmation to reduce defensiveness prior to persuasion attempts (Sherman and Cohen 2006).

Scientific expertise, training in research methods and rational thinking

Increasing people's knowledge of research methodology and statistical reasoning through graduate training can increase people's ability to use statistical and methodological reasoning about everyday life events (Nisbett et al. 1987; Lehman et al. 1988). Such improvements in reasoning could also decrease the risk of science denial. In support of this hypothesis, experienced scientists show an increased ability to reject hypotheses in response to disconfirming evidence (Dunbar 1995). Unfortunately, it seems that scientific reasoning skills are not a 'cure all' for science denial. For example, science comprehension is unrelated to people's assessments of climate change risk (Kahan 2013).

Group-level mechanisms leading to science denial

Although most psychological research has focused on individual-level causes of science denial, individual-level explanations are only a part of the picture. Recent studies suggest that group-level processes may also play a key role in science denial (Kahan et al. 2010; Lewandowsky et al. 2013d; Nauroth et al. 2014). This section reviews findings in two core areas: (1) social identity processes and (2) ideology, cultural values, and cultural cognition.

Social identity processes

According to social identity theory (Tajfel and Turner 1986), individuals have personal identities (differentiating the self from others) and social identities based on group memberships (differentiating 'us' from 'them'). Ingroup favoritism is a key feature of social identification (Brewer 2007). When a valued social identity is threatened, group members may respond with anger and hostility, protect the ingroup, and aggress against the threat (Ellemers et al. 2002; McCoy and Major 2003).

An area of science denial in which social identity may play a key role is the anti-vaccine movement. For instance, Hoffman and colleagues (2019) found that Facebook serves as an effective platform for anti-vaccine groups to form and spread harmful denial messages (e.g., 'poliovirus does not exist' and 'pesticides caused clinical symptoms of polio'). Such messages are most likely to be influential if posted by ingroup members while opposing views from outgroup members are likely to be denied. For instance, preliminary experimental evidence suggests that priming social identity among members of the anti-vaccine community increases science denial of research showing vaccine safety, especially among highly identified group members (Prot et al. 2019).

Ideology, cultural values, and cultural cognition

Ideology and cultural worldviews also play a role in science denial. For instance, free-market ideology predicts rejection of climate science as well as rejection of other well-supported scientific findings (e.g., effects of smoking on lung cancer and effects of HIV on AIDS; Lewandowsky et al. 2012, 2013a, d).

Cultural cognition affects not only what people believe but also whom they believe. In a study by Kahan and colleagues (2010), participants were more likely to view experts as credible and to be persuaded by them if they believed that the experts shared their cultural values. For example, when a hierarchical and individualistic expert defended the HPV vaccine as safe, participants who shared those values were more likely to adopt a more positive attitude towards the vaccine. Egalitarian participants were more easily persuaded by an egalitarian expert.

This line of research provides the basis for developing more effective methods of science communication. It suggests that persuasion attempts will be most effective when information is presented in ways that affirm people's cultural values and ideologies instead of threatening them (Cohen et al. 2000, 2007). It also helps to involve a diverse set of experts as public advocates, ensuring that within the set at least one expert is viewed as credible by people with different worldviews (Kahan et al. 2010).

Intergroup processes leading to science denial

An intergroup perspective may be especially useful when searching for the roots of angry denial and aggression towards scientists. At first, the anger and hostile behaviors that often go hand-in-hand with science denial may seem puzzling. However, these emotional reactions and behaviors are no longer surprising when considered from an intergroup conflict perspective. Among some denialists, scientists are viewed as a hostile outgroup that derogates and threatens the ingroup (Lewandowsky et al. 2013a; Nauroth et al. 2014).

Two theoretical perspectives from the area of intergroup conflict are discussed which offer valuable insights into possible origins of angry science denial and aggression towards scientists: (1) intergroup emotions theory and (2) intergroup threat theory.

Intergroup emotions theory

When social identity is salient, group-relevant events elicit intergroup emotions (e.g., football fans experiencing elation after their team wins; see Mackie et al. 2000). Highly identified group members experience and express stronger group emotions.

Group-level emotions are shared within the ingroup—people's emotions converge towards those prototypical of their group (Smith et al. 2007). Strength of group-level emotions depends on the level of social identification. People who are highly identified with the ingroup tend to experience and express stronger group emotions than weak identifiers (Smith et al. 2007). For example, in the area of science denial, Nauroth and colleagues (2014) found that strongly identified video gamers experienced greater anger in response to research showing video game violence increases aggression, suggesting that this may be a group-level emotion. Prot and colleagues (2019) found greater feelings of distrust towards vaccine researchers among strongly identified members of the anti-vaccine community.

Group-level emotions motivate and regulate intergroup attitudes and behaviors (Mackie et al. 2000; Smith et al. 2007). Different types of ingroup and outgroup appraisals lead to different emotions, causing different behaviors towards outgroups (Mackie et al. 2000). For example, when an outgroup is appraised as threatening, this elicits distinct emotional responses—fear leading to avoidance of the outgroup or anger leading to confrontation (Mackie and Smith 2014).

Intergroup emotions theory (Mackie et al. 2000; Mackie and Smith 2014) provides a valuable conceptual framework for understanding angry science denial. When emotional reactions that denialists express towards research findings and researchers are examined at an individual level, distinct emotional responses can be difficult to explain. It would seem surprising that denialists have heated emotional reactions to research findings and public policy that have no impact on them personally. Intergroup emotions theory suggests a clear explanation—research and researchers should engender such responses if they influence one's valued ingroup.

Intergroup threat theory

When ingroup members perceive that outgroup members are in a position to harm them, they experience intergroup threat (Stephan and Stephan 2000; Stephan et al. 2002). Realistic threats jeopardize the physical or material well-being of the ingroup. In contrast, symbolic threats endanger the ingroup worldview. They arise from perceived group differences in morals, values, standards, beliefs, and attitudes (Stephan et al. 2002). Intergroup threat theory is compatible with the framework of intergroup emotions theory and contributes to predicting discrete emotional reactions towards outgroups (Cottrell and Neuberg 2005). For instance, physical and safety threats tend to predict fear and contamination threats predict disgust, whereas threats to freedom predict anger.

It is likely that intergroup threat plays a key role in angry science denial. Preliminary experimental findings show that perceived threat from scientists increases science denial, anger, and aggressive intentions (Prot et al. 2019). The type of threat perceived by denialists is likely to differ between groups. For example, parents who oppose vaccinations may view vaccines and pro-vaccine researchers as a realistic threat to their children's health and safety (Hoffman et al. 2019).

Conclusive thoughts

Doubt and denial of scientific evidence in areas such as vaccination safety, dangers of tobacco use, and effectiveness of HIV prevention strategies lead to detrimental outcomes both to individuals and to our society. It might seem hard to understand why such denial persists in the face of clear evidence and scientific consensus and why it is often accompanied by anger and aggression towards scientists. Science denial is a complex phenomenon that is influenced by a number of individual-level, group-level, and intergroup processes. Understanding the complex set of factors causing science denial can help develop more effective intervention strategies to combat science denial and bolster trust in science-based medical practices.

Research on psychological mechanisms of science denial offers a basis for developing effective prevention and intervention strategies. Several studies on individual-level causes of science denial point to effective ways of combating belief perseverance, including discussing the perseverance process with participants (Ross et al. 1975), manipulating self-awareness (Davies 1982), and prompting participants to consider the opposite position (Lord et al. 1984) or to generate causal theories in both possible directions (Anderson 1983). Self-affirmation through bolstering a valued self-image has been found to lower defensiveness and promote responsiveness to health messages such as smokers' reactions to graphic cigarette warning labels (Harris et al. 2007) and women's acceptance of warnings of cancer risk from their alcohol consumption (Harris and Napper 2005). Importantly, self-affirmation has also been effective in promoting positive health behaviors (Sherman et al. 2000). Self-affirmation and priming attachment thoughts and memories could provide quick and effective ways to lower the risk of health messages causing boomerang effects (such as those observed by Nyhan et al. 2014).

When science denial is bolstered by group-level and intergroup-level factors, interventions targeting group- and intergroup-level causes may be more effective. For instance, to combat vaccine myths spread among the anti-vaccine communities via Facebook, Hoffman et al. (2019) have prompted health professionals to use social networks to deliver targeted messages to different groups at risk. Interventions aimed at reducing intergroup conflict could be especially helpful when trust in the scientific community is low and scientists are instead viewed as a hostile group. Such interventions could help lower fear and anger towards scientists, lowering risk of harassment towards scientists carrying out controversial research (Lewandowsky et al. 2013c).

References

Anderson CA (1983) Abstract and concrete data in the perseverance of social theories: when weak data lead to unshakeable beliefs. *Journal of Experimental Social Psychology* 19:93–108

Anderson CA and Kellam KL (1992) Belief perseverance, biased assimilation, and covariation detection: the effects of hypothetical social theories and new data. *Personality and Social Psychology Bulletin* 18:555–565

Anderson CA, Lepper MR and Ross L (1980) The perseverance of social theories: the role of explanation in the persistence of discredited information. *Journal of Personality and Social Psychology* 39:1037–1049

Anderson CA, New BL and Speer JR (1985) Argument availability as a mediator of social theory perseverance. *Social Cognition* 3:235–249

Atwell JE, Van Otterloo J, Zipprich J, Winter K, Harriman K, Salmon DA, Halsey NA and Omer SB (2013) Nonmedical vaccine exemptions and pertussis in California, 2010. *Pediatrics* 132(4):624–630

Bateman C (2007) Paying the price for AIDS denialism. *South African Medical Journal* 97:912–914

Bogart LM, Kalichman SC and Simbayi LC (2008) Endorsement of a genocidal HIV conspiracy as a barrier to HIV testing in South Africa. *Journal of Acquired Immune Deficiency Syndromes* 49(1):115–116

Brehm SS and Brehm JW (1981) *Psychological reactance*. New York: Wiley

Brewer MB (2007) The social psychology of intergroup relations: social categorization, ingroup bias, and outgroup prejudice. In Kruglanski AW and Higgins ET (eds.) *Social psychology: handbook of basic principles*. New York: Guilford Press

Cohen GL, Aronson J and Steele CM (2000) When beliefs yield to evidence: reducing biased evaluation by affirming the self. *Personality and Social Psychology Bulletin* 26:1151–1164

Cohen GL, Sherman DK, Bastardi A, McGoey M, Hsu A and Ross L (2007) Bridging the partisan divide: self-affirmation reduces ideological closed-mindedness and inflexibility in negotiation. *Journal of Personality and Social Psychology* 93:415–430

Cottrell CA and Neuberg SL (2005) Different emotional reactions to different groups: a sociofunctional threat-based approach to 'prejudice.' *Journal of Personality & Social Psychology* 88:770–789

Davies MF (1982) Self-focused attention and belief perseverance. Journal of Experimental Social Psychology 18:595–605

Deer B (2004) Revealed: MMR research scandal. *The Sunday Times*. Available at: http://briandeer.com/mmr/lancet-deer-1.htm

Diethelm P and McKee M (2009) Denialism: what is it and how should scientists respond? *European Journal of Public Health* 19:2–4

Dunbar K (1995) How scientists really reason: scientific reasoning in real-world laboratories. In Sternberg RJ and Davidson JE (eds.) *Mechanisms of insight*. Cambridge: MIT Press

The Editors of the Lancet (2010) Retraction – Ileal-lymphoid-nodular hyperplasia, non-specific colitis, and pervasive developmental disorder in children. *The Lancet* 375(9713):445

Ellemers N, Spears R and Doosje B (2002) Self and social identity. In Fiske ST, Schacter DL and Zahn-Waxler C (eds.) *Annual review of psychology*, vol. 53. Palo Alto, CA: Annual Reviews

Feather NT (1962) Cigarette smoking and lung cancer: a study of cognitive dissonance. *Australian Journal of Psychology* 14:55–64

Feather NT (1963) Cognitive dissonance, sensitivity, and evaluation. *Journal of Abnormal and Social Psychology* 66:157–163

Festinger LA (1957) *A theory of cognitive dissonance*. Evanston, IL: Row, Peterson

The Flat Earth Society (2019) History of the flat earth society. Available at: http://theflatearthsociety.org/cms/index.php/about-the-society/history-and-mission

Gerber JS and Offit PA (2009) Vaccines and autism: a tale of shifting hypotheses. *Clinical Infectious Diseases* 48(4):456–461

Gibbons FX, Eggleston TJ and Benthin AC (1997) Cognitive reactions to smoking relapse: the reciprocal relation between dissonance and self-esteem. *Journal of Personality and Social Psychology* 72(1):184–195

Gibbons FX, McGovern PG and Lando HA (1991) Relapse and risk perception among members of a smoking cessation clinic. *Health Psychology* 10:42–45

Harris PR, Mayle K, Mabbott L and Napper L (2007) Self-affirmation reduces smokers' defensiveness to graphic on-pack cigarette warning labels. *Health Psychology* 26:437–446

Harris PR and Napper L (2005) Self-affirmation and the biased processing of threatening health-risk information. *Personality and Social Psychology Bulletin* 31:1250–1263

Hart PS and Nisbet EC (2011) Boomerang effects in science communication: how motivated reasoning and identity cues amplify opinion polarization about climate mitigation policies. *Communication Research* 39(6):701–723

Hoffman BL, Felter EM, Chu K, Shensa A, Hermann C, Wolynn T, Williams D and Primack BA (2019) It's not all about autism: the emerging landscape of anti-vaccination sentiment on Facebook. *Vaccine* 37(16):22216–2223

Jacques PJ (2012) A general theory of climate denial. *Global Environmental Politics* 12:9–17

Johnson RE (1968) Smoking and the reduction of cognitive dissonance. *Journal of Personality and Social Psychology* 9:260–265

Kahan DM (2013) Making climate-science communication evidence-based – all the way down. In Boykoff M and Crow D (eds.) *Culture, politics and climate change*. Oxon: Routledge Press

Kahan DM, Braman D, Cohen G, Slovic P and Gastil J (2010) Who fears the HPV vaccine, who doesn't, and why: an experimental study of the mechanisms of cultural cognition. *Law and Human Behavior* 34(6):501–516

Klayman J and Ha YW (1987) Confirmation, disconfirmation, and information in hypotheses testing. *Psychological Review* 94:211–228

Kleiman T and Hassin RR (2013) When conflicts are good: nonconscious goal conflicts reduce confirmatory thinking. *Journal of Personality and Social Psychology* 105(3):374–387

Landman A and Glantz SA (2009) Tobacco industry efforts to undermine policy-relevant research. *American Journal of Public Health* 99:45–58

Lawton MP and Goldman AE (1961) Cigarette smoking and attitude toward the etiology of lung cancer. *Journal of Social Psychology* 54:235–248

Lehman DR, Lampert RO and Nisbett RE (1988) The effects of graduate training on reasoning: formal discipline and thinking about everyday-life. *American Psychologist* 43(6):431–442

Lewandowsky S, Cook J, Oberauer K and Marriott M (2013a) Recursive fury: conspiracist ideation in the blogosphere in response to research on conspiracist ideation. Available at: www.psychology.uwa.edu.au/__data/assets/pdf_file/0003/2523540/LskyetalRecursive-Fury4UWA.pdf

Lewandowsky S, Ecker UKH, Seifert C, Schwarz N and Cook J (2012) Misinformation and its correction: continued influence and successful debiasing. *Psychological Science in the Public Interest* 13:106–131

Lewandowsky S, Gignac GE and Oberauer K (2013b) The role of conspiracist ideation and worldviews in predicting rejection of science. *PloS1* 8(10):e75637

Lewandowsky S, Mann ME, Bauld L, Hastings G and Loftus EF (2013c) The subterranean war on Science. *The Observer (Association for Psychological Science)*. Available at: www.psychologicalscience.org/index.php/publications/observer/2013/november-2013/the-subterranean-war-on-science.html

Lewandowsky S, Oberauer K and Gignac GE (2013d) NASA faked the moon landing – therefore, (climate) science is a hoax: an anatomy of the motivated rejection of science. *Psychological Science* 24(5):622–633

Lord CG, Lepper MR and Preston E (1984) Considering the opposite: a corrective strategy for social judgment. *Journal of Personality and Social Psychology* 47:1231–1243

Lord CG, Ross L and Lepper MR (1979) Biased assimilation and attitude polarization: the effects of prior theories on subsequently considered evidence. *Journal of Personality and Social Psychology* 37(11):2098–2109

Mackie DM, Devos T and Smith ER (2000) Intergroup emotions: explaining offensive action tendencies in an intergroup context. *Journal of Personality and Social Psychology* 79(4):602–616

Mackie DM and Smith ER (2014) Intergroup emotions. In Dovidio J and Simpson J (eds.) *APA handbook of personality and social psychology* (Volume II: Interpersonal Relationships and Group Processes). Washington, DC: APA Press

Maglione MA, Das L, Raaen L, Smith A, Chari R, Newberry S, Perry T, Bidwell Goetz M and Gidengil C (2014) Safety of vaccines used for routine immunization of US children: a systematic review. *Pediatrics* 134(2)

McCoy S and Major B (2003) Group identification moderates emotional responses to perceived prejudice. *Personality and Social Psychology Bulletin* 29(8):1005–1017

McFarland C, Cheam A and Buehler R (2007) The perseverance effect in the debriefing paradigm: replication and extension. *Journal of Experimental Social Psychology* 43:233–240

Morris KA and Swann WB (1996) Denial and the AIDS crisis: on wishing away the threat of AIDS. In Oskamp S and Thompson S (eds.) *Safer sex in the '90s: understanding and preventing HIV risk behavior*. New York: Sage

Nature (2010) Science subpoenaed. *Nature* 46:135–136

Nauroth P, Gollwitzer M, Bender J and Rothmund T (2014) Gamers against science: the case of the violent video games debate. *European Journal of Social Psychology* 44(2):104–116

Nisbett RE, Fong GT, Lehman DR and Cheng PW (1987) Teaching reasoning. *Science* 238:625–631

Nyhan B, Reifler J, Richey S and Freed GL (2014) Effective messages in vaccine promotion: a randomized trial. *Pediatrics* 33:e835

Pervin LA and Yatko RJ (1965) Cigarette smoking and alternative methods of reducing dissonance. *Journal of Personality and Social Psychology* 2:30–36

Poland GA and Spier R (2010) Fear, misinformation, and innumerates: how the Wakefield paper, the press, and advocacy groups damaged the public health. *Vaccine* 28(12):2361–2362

Prot S, Anderson CA, Blankenship KB, Gentile DG, Krizan Z and Saleem M (2019) Science denial as intergroup conflict: using social identity theory, intergroup emotions theory and intergroup threat theory to explain angry denial of science. [Manuscript in preparation]

Reed MB and Aspinwall LG (1998) Self-affirmation reduces biased processing of health-risk information. *Motivation and Emotion* 22:99–132

Ross L, Lepper MR and Hubbard M (1975) Perseverance in self-perception and social perception: biased attributional processes in the debriefing paradigm. *Journal of Personality and Social Psychology* 32:880–892

Saleem M, Prot S, Cikara M, Lam BCP, Anderson CA and Jelic M (2015) Cutting Gordian knots: reducing prejudice through attachment security. *Personality and Social Psychology Bulletin* 41:1560–1574

Sherman DAK, Nelson LD and Steele CM (2000) Do messages about health risks threaten the self? Increasing the acceptance of threatening health messages via self-affirmation. *Personality and Social Psychology Bulletin* 26(9):1046–1058

Sherman DK and Cohen JL (2006) The psychology of self-defense: self-affirmation theory. In Zanna MP (ed.) *Advances in experimental social psychology*, vol. 38. San Diego, CA: Academic Press

Smith ER, Seger CR and Mackie DM (2007) Can emotions be truly group level? Evidence regarding four conceptual criteria. *Journal of Personality and Social Psychology* 93(3):431–446

Stanovich KE and West RF (2008) On the failure of intelligence to predict myside bias and one-sided bias. *Thinking & Reasoning* 14:129–167

Stanovich KE, West RF and Toplak ME (2013) Myside bias, rational thinking, and intelligence. *Current Directions in Psychological Science* 22:259–264

Stephan W and Stephan CW (2000) An integrated threat theory of prejudice. In Oskamp S (ed.) *Reducing prejudice and discrimination*. Hillsdale, NJ: Erlbaum

Stephan WG, Boniecki KA, Ybarra O, Bettencourt A, Ervin KS, Jackson LA, McNatt P and Renfro L (2002) The role of threats in the racial attitudes of Blacks and Whites. *Personality and Social Psychology Bulletin* 28:1242–1254

Sugerman DE, Barskey AE, Delea MG, Ortega-Sanchez IR, Bi D, Ralston KJ, Rota PA, Waters-Montijo K and Lebaron CW (2010) Measles outbreak in a highly vaccinated population, San Diego, 2008: role of the intentionally undervaccinated. *Pediatrics* 125(4):747–755

Tajfel H and Turner JC (1986) The social identity theory of inter-group behavior. In Worchel S and Austin LW (eds.) *The psychology of intergroup relations*. Chicago: Nelson-Hall, pp. 7–24

Taylor B, Miller E, Farrington CP, Petropoulos MC, Favot-Mayaud I, Li J and Waight PA (1999) Autism and measles, mumps, and rubella vaccine: no epidemiological evidence for a causal association. *Lancet* 353:2026–2029

Wakefield AJ, Murch SH, Anthony A, Linnell J, Casson DM, Malik M, Dhillon AP, Thomson MA, Harvey P, Valentine A, Davies SE and Walker-Smith JE (1998) Ileal-lymphoid-nodular hyperplasia, non-specific colitis, and pervasive developmental disorder in children. *Lancet* 351:637–641

Willemsen MC and De Zwart W (1999) The effectiveness of policy and health education strategies for reducing adolescent smoking: a review of the evidence. *Journal of Adolescence* 22(5):587–599

4 Understanding the demand for illicit lifestyle medicines online

An analysis of the risk perception of consumers

Rosa Koenraadt

Introduction

In recent years, the purchase of all sorts of legal, semi-legal, and illicit medicines online has increased steadily (Evans-Brown et al. 2012; WHO 2012; Di Nicola et al. 2015; Hall and Antonopoulos 2016; Koenraadt and de Haan 2016). A particular concern is the *illicit* trade in medicines online: on a wide variety of websites such as illegal online pharmacies and secondhand vending sites, all sorts of counterfeit or otherwise illicit medicines can be easily purchased without a medical prescription or medical oversight (Evans-Brown et al. 2012; WHO 2012; Di Nicola et al. 2015; Hall and Antonopoulos 2016; Koenraadt and de Haan 2016; Koenraadt and van de Ven 2017). Illicit medicines can contain effective ingredients; however, they can also be contaminated by hazardous substances or contain no active ingredients at all. As a result, patients or other consumers cannot be certain that the active ingredients, side effects, and medical outcome will match what appears on the label (Fernandez et al. 2008; Venhuis et al. 2011; WHO 2012).

As the consumption of illicit medicines is thus associated with various health risks, and the demand for illicit medicines seems to be on the rise, it is important to provide effective health messages that inform consumers on the potential risks of ordering medicines outside the official supply chain online. In the literature, the focus generally lies on the deceived consumers and how they unwittingly may purchase fraudulent medicines (WHO 2012; Blackstone et al. 2014). However, some consumer groups may also deliberately purchase illicit medicines online for nonmedical use of medical products (Evans-Brown et al. 2012). In essence, consumers may purchase illicit medicines online for different reasons, and thus evaluate medical information and risks differently. In order to design effective health policies for all consumers, it is important to better understand distinctive motives and risk perceptions of consumers who purchase (potentially harmful) medicines without medical oversight online. This chapter focuses on the consumers of illicit lifestyle medicines (with a specific focus on erectile dysfunction and weight loss products) and offers an analysis into their motives, perceptions, and risk management strategies.

As the internet is increasingly used for selling and purchasing illicit medicines, consumers continue to be prone to buying potentially harmful products online. Similar to medical treatments and wellness approaches that are developed outside science-based medicine and that are widely advertised online (see, for instance, chapters 8 and 9), the quality and effectiveness of many illicit medicines sold online is not guaranteed. As such, without this warranty users have to evaluate the information, quality, safety, and efficacy of the medical products by themselves. It is therefore key to understand how and why consumers turn to the internet, how online information on medicines is evaluated, and how the risks of retrieving misleading medical information or harmful products are perceived by them. This understanding can help us to better comprehend various types of potentially dangerous health-related behaviours online, including the ones explored in other chapters on this book.

Background

Generally speaking, in western countries the whole chain of medicines (from production to consumption) is strictly regulated at both the national and international levels. In recent years, however, it has been suggested that a global trade in all sorts of falsified and otherwise illicit medicines (such as counterfeit, adulterated, and unlicensed drugs) is flourishing (Evans-Brown et al. 2012; WHO 2012; Di Nicola et al. 2015; Hall and Antonopoulos 2016; Koenraadt and de Haan 2016). In this study, the umbrella term of illicit medicines will be used, which includes all medicines that are not produced, traded, or sold according to national or international regulations, regardless of the level in the supply chain where the infringement takes place (see also Hall and Antonopoulos 2016; Koenraadt 2018).

Most illicit medicines reaching western countries are traded online. The range of these medicines is diverse and includes lifestyle medicines such as erectile dysfunction products, slimming pills, pain killers, antiviral medication, antidepressants, and antibiotics, as well as a wide range of narcotic analgesics, stimulants, and benzodiazepines (Orizio et al. 2011; Lavorgna 2014). In the online world, there is limited control over the sale of these illicit medicines, which means that there can be a degree of uncertainty over what the consumer is actually purchasing (Orizio et al. 2011; Venhuis et al. 2011). Indeed, digital technologies have had an important influence on the purchase and consumption of medicines. Patients and consumers can easily look up all sorts of medical information online: they can check the symptoms of certain pathologies, their modes of prevention, as well as use self-diagnosis tests and online platforms for discussions with fellow patients (Nettleton 2013). The vast array of medical advice and information that can be accessed online has led to both positive and negative reactions, with some being concerned over the possibility of being misled by wrong information, while others emphasise the empowering potential of online medical information (Nettleton and Hanlon 2006; Nettleton 2013).

As both licit and illicit medicines can be offered online, it is not always clear to the user which medical product he or she is purchasing. For example, medicines could generally be sold on the legal market where the products are manufactured, distributed, and sold through the licensed and regulated supply chain. This includes medicines available on prescription through a legitimate online pharmacy. At the same time, a growing illicit market exists where unapproved supplements and unlicensed lifestyle medicines are being sold. This includes the sale of counterfeit medicines or unlicensed generics (Venhuis et al. 2011). Furthermore, a 'grey' market for lifestyle medicines can be identified, which mainly refers to (potentially adulterated) food supplements with experimental chemical substances. Because experimental substances are often unknown, these products generally do not (yet) fall under medicine or food legislation of national countries (Venhuis et al. 2009, 2011).

The online trade in illicit medicines is often believed to use anonymity as a major marketing strategy. This plays straight into consumer motivations, such as the embarrassment of purchasing sexual enhancing medicines (Intomart 2009, 2012). Since an important, yet unknown, share of the medicines sold online are considered falsified or otherwise illicit, the risk of illegal pharmacies using deceptive marketing claims is high (WHO 2012; IRACM 2013). With blurring boundaries between what is legal and what is illegal in the online environment, and given the improved techniques for falsifying medicines, packages, and online logos of official trademarks, consumers might not even realise that they are purchasing illicit medicines (Lavorgna 2014; Di Nicola et al. 2015).

This applies particularly to the increasing online availability of illicit 'lifestyle medicines' that often lie at the intersection of legal and illegal medicine markets. Lifestyle medicines can be defined as medicines that could modify or change nonmedical or non-health-related goals or conditions that lie at the margins of health and wellbeing (Gilbert et al. 2000; Rahman et al. 2010). While most lifestyle medicines are available through official sources for particular purposes and often require a prescription, they are also taken for non-authorised reasons to improve someone's life, physical function, or appearance. In case these medicines are sold on the illicit market and primarily used for recreational reasons, lifestyle medicines are also often referred to as human enhancement drugs (McVeigh et al. 2012). This includes sexual enhancers, muscle drugs, or cognitive enhancers, which are often used for recreational purposes. In these instances, the lifestyle medicines are taken to improve bodily, mental, and sexual capabilities, as opposed to curing or managing an illness.

Although the exact prevalence of these substances is unknown, in recent years legal and illegal lifestyle drugs are in high demand (Evans-Brown et al. 2012; Brennan et al. 2013; Koenraadt and Van de Ven 2017). However, there is limited information available on distinct groups of consumers that actually purchase illicit lifestyle medicines and how they evaluate the notion of risk online. In most studies, there is no differentiation between medicines bought legally or illegally online, between the types of consumers, between medicines bought wittingly or unwittingly, and between the types of medicines purchased on the internet—although these may greatly vary across the types of consumers. In order to design effective health policies for all, it is vital to distinguish among different types of consumers and how they evaluate risks and the quality of online medical information. In this chapter, the focus lies on the demand side of the online market for lifestyle medicines, with a particular focus on medicines for erectile dysfunction and weight loss. After providing a classification of different types of consumers purchasing illicit medicines online, I analyse how these consumer groups perceive the risks of buying medicines online in an effort to elucidate how trust and risk can be differently evaluated by them in the online world.

Methods

This chapter is based on the author's doctoral study on the demand and supply of illicit weight loss medicines and sexual enhancers in the Netherlands (see Koenraadt (2018) for a detailed description of the methodology). This study was conducted between January 2014 and August 2015, and a multi-method approach was used, including the use of quantitative and qualitative data sources. For the purpose of this chapter, the following methods are relevant. First, data from 81 semi-structured interviews with officials (N = 39), suppliers (N = 32), and consumers (N = 32) have been used. Participants were recruited on- and offline, via telephone, by visiting relevant markets and shops such as supplement stores and sex shops, and through a snowballing method whereby existing participants introduced new interlocutors. Second, an analysis of discussion platforms and 17 websites that were used to sell and trade illicit weight loss drugs and sexual enhancers was conducted. Third, quantitative data were obtained through a survey study in the Netherlands: a prevalence study was conducted among a panel of 50,848 Dutch respondents, after which an in-depth study among 985 consumers of illicit medicines took place; the in-depth study included 447 respondents that purchased illicit medicines online and consisted of 60 questions divided into various themes, such as purchasing behaviour, satisfaction, motivations, and risk perception (see also Koenraadt and de Haan 2016). A total of 88 respondents purchased sexual enhancers, while 77 consumers purchased weight loss drugs.

Data was analysed by means of open coding through the software program NVivo. Utrecht University's Faculty of Law, Economics and Government granted ethical approval for the study.

Results

Classifying online purchasers of illicit medicines

In order to understand the risk perception of purchasers of online lifestyle medicines, first it is important to distinguish the motivations of why consumers turn to the internet to purchase these products: users can in fact have medical or recreational reasons for the consumption of illicit medicines. In addition, they can be deceived into buying them, or deliberately do so. Therefore, various analytical subgroups can be identified, with a distinction between deceived and non-deceived, and between medical and nonmedical consumers (Figure 4.1).

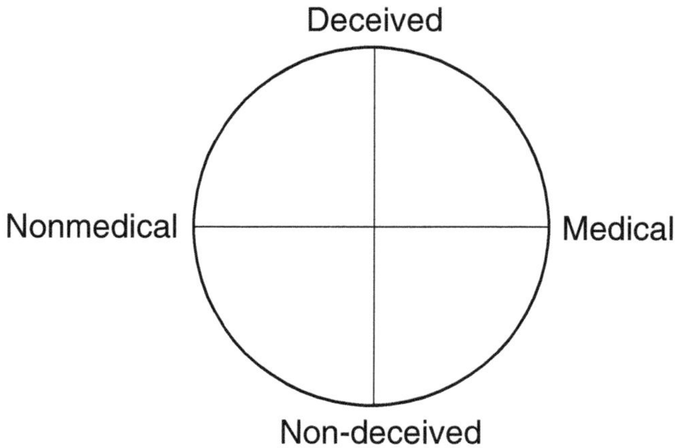

Figure 4.1 Classification of consumers of illicit medicines

Medical consumers

Medical consumers turn to the online market for illicit lifestyle medicines for different reasons. More than half of the respondents of our survey study who purchased illicit lifestyle medicines online mentioned convenience as an important motivator (see also Koenraadt and de Haan 2016). Respondents primarily referred to the possibility of ordering medicines at any given moment, outside office hours, and receiving them directly at home: with just a couple of mouse clicks, all sorts of medicines can be accessed, compared and ordered, and sent by mail to a home address, thus circumventing waiting lines and office hours (in line with Di Nicola et al. 2015). In addition, both the quantitative survey and the in-depth interviews conducted suggest that financial considerations are among the primary reasons that lead customers turn to the internet for medicines. Online sources enable potential medical consumers to compare prices, content, and reviews, after which they may choose to purchase the cheapest available option (see also Bessell et al. 2003; Di Nicola et al. 2015; Hall and Antonopoulos 2016). In a study on unauthorised online pharmacies, consumers explained that medicines were cheaper compared to local pharmacies because of fewer regulatory restrictions (Ivanitskaya et al. 2010).

In line with existing studies (Bessell et al. 2003; Nicolosi et al. 2006; Orizio and Gelatti 2010; Di Nicola et al. 2015; Hall and Antonopoulos 2016), my analysis shows that shame and embarrassment are also important drivers. This also coincides with findings that men are reluctant to seek medical care for sexual problems (see, for instance, Gott and Hinchliff 2003; Moreira et al. 2005). Sexual enhancers are the lifestyle medicines that are most directly associated with embarrassment and, based on our survey, 24% of the consumers of sexual enhancers reported that they purchased medicines online because they did not want to discuss their condition with a doctor. Purchasing medicines through unofficial sources generally enables patients to avoid both the time and hassle of a doctor's appointment and the awkward face-to-face conversations that might be expected there (Gott and Hinchliff 2003; Philaretou 2004).

Recreational consumers

If convenience, financial concerns, and the desire to avoid embarrassment may stimulate primarily medical consumers to purchase illicit lifestyle medicines online, different reasons motivate recreational consumers to turn to the internet to purchase their products of choice. Indeed, recreational consumers want to buy medicines that are not available in the Netherlands, or purchase prescription-only medicines without having a prescription. Recreational (or nonmedical) consumers of lifestyle medicines include, for instance, bodybuilders who use steroids to increase muscle mass (Monaghan 2001; Paoli and Donati 2014; Van de Ven 2016), students who use cognitive enhancers such as Ritalin for better study results (Mazanov et al. 2013), or consumers who take sexual enhancers (e.g., Viagra) to improve their night life (Intomart 2009, 2012; Koenraadt 2012; Evans-Brown et al. 2012; Koenraadt and de Haan 2016). In most of these instances, users consume products that are not legally sold or whose consumption would not be recommended to them by a doctor. As such, these consumers resort to the online world to obtain their drug of choice.

Illicit medicine consumption for nonmedical purposes was found abundantly in this research. Almost all interviewed retailers confirmed that their consumers tend to purchase sexual enhancers for a recreational use or weight loss. These findings are consistent with those gathered in other studies, which emphasise the recreational consumption of sexual enhancers in all sorts of recreational settings. For example, the recreational use of prescription medicines for sexual enhancement is reportedly used in combination with drugs or alcohol, primarily in night-life settings (Bechara et al. 2010; Benschop et al. 2011). Curiosity and peer pressure contribute to decisions to use medical sexual enhancers also in non-socio-recreational settings (Musacchio et al. 2006; Peters et al. 2007; Apodaca and Moser 2011)—the aim is to gain extra confidence or prestige or to seek for experimentation. Similarly, while prescriptions for weight loss medicines are intended for people whose health is at risk if they do not lose weight, various interview respondents have explained their use of strong weight loss medication not available in the Netherlands for lifestyle and physical appearance purposes. For instance, these products can be used to get extra energy, which is a side effect of appetite-reducing medicines. As such, a significant group of illicit medicine consumers take medicines for no reason beyond enhancement, lifestyle, or recreational purposes; the medical foundations for the drugs they take have no place in their decision-making process.

Deceived vs non-deceived consumers

Whereas various medical or recreational motives may stimulate consumers to purchase medicines through online sources, a second distinction can be made between consumers who may be under the impression they are buying legal medicines and others who deliberately purchase them through illicit sources online. Heinonen and colleagues (2014) argue that a distinction should be made between deceptive and non-deceptive counterfeit products: whereas *deceived* consumers are not aware of the fact they are purchasing fake or illicit products, the *non-deceived* consumers understand exactly what they are doing—although they might not have a clear understanding of how the risks of their choices should be evaluated. This distinction is highly visible in the entire illicit medicine market, but is sharpest among customers who buy via the internet.

Deceived consumers are misled into purchasing illicit products. In cyberspace, this is due to the fact that the quality of health information and medicines purchased online is rarely guaranteed and, as such, consumers may experience difficulties in determining the genuineness of an online supplier and quality of its products (in line with previous research, such as Jackson et al. 2010; Di Giorgio 2011; Gaudiono et al. 2012; IRACM 2013). For example, several studies have shown that often online pharmacies do not mention the risks of taking specific medicines, that limited medical information is listed, or that inaccurate information is provided (Bessell et al. 2003; Wassink et al. 2010). In addition, online pharmacies may provide prescription medicines without requiring the customer to present a prescription. Sometimes, an online questionnaire is used to give the customer the perception that the online pharmacy is engaging in a rigorous medical analysis as a substitute for a doctor's prescription (Orizio et al. 2011). When purchasing medicines online, consumers are thus not always aware that they are being deceived (Montoya and Jano 2007; Orizio et al. 2011). Images of doctors in white coats, a professional presentation, and fake diagnosis tests can create an impression that all the medicines offered by these sites are legal. Professional website designs cover untrustworthy features and mimic reputable contribute to purposely mislead consumers (Ivanitskaya et al. 2010). The widespread availability of all sorts of information and distribution channels on the surface web challenges consumers who wish to determine the legitimacy of online pharmacies (Lavorgna 2014; Di Nicola et al. 2015).

On the contrary, such concerns are not relevant to consumers who are aware they are purchasing medicines through unofficial routes. These customers believe they understand the risks inherent in purchasing medicines outside official distribution chains, but these are outweighed by motivations such as convenience, finance, or embarrassment. For instance, recreational consumers are generally well aware that they are using medicines for purposes that are beyond the scope supported by the Dutch medical establishment, and they know that official providers would refuse to sell these pharmaceuticals to them. However, also nonmedical consumers can be deceived into purchasing illicit medicines, for example, by not knowing that a prescription is needed.

Risk perception online

In order to understand the risk perception of the online consumers, it is important to distinguish among the main reasons for consumption—whether it be

Table 4.1 Reasons why buyers trust a website when purchasing illicit medicines online ($n = 153$)

	Sexual enhancers (N = 88) (%)	*Weight loss medicines (N = 70) (%)*
Clear information about vendor and medicine	42	43
Clear overview of available medicines	35	25
Reviews of others	26	44
Vendor's expertise	5	7
I know the vendor	6	3
Other	24	6

Source: Analysis of own survey data

medical or recreational (and everything in between)—and whether users deliberately turn to illicit sources or not. In this section, the risk perceptions of different types of consumers of illicit medicines is further outlined, with a particular focus on the *non-deceived recreational consumers* of illicit lifestyle medicines.

In all medical contexts, trust is fundamental: patients have to believe that health care professionals direct all their knowledge to serve patients' best interests (Hall et al. 2001). However, the supplier/consumer relationships of health products in an online context are very peculiar, and specific mechanisms are used to establish, develop, and maintain trust. Overall, our survey data show that consumers have generally high levels of trust in the websites they employ for purchasing illicit lifestyle medicines. As presented in Table 4.1, clear information about the vendor and available medicines, such as reviews of others, are the most important factors that buyers take into account when purchasing lifestyle medicines online.

Some internet consumers claim they are able to evaluate the quality of the medicines they purchase. Based on the survey, it appears that 24% of the 153 consumers consider themselves very well capable of identifying the trustworthiness of the website, and 18% of them are well capable of estimating the quality of online purchased medicines. This applies particularly for the group of *deceived consumers* who overall have good faith and belief in the medical information they retrieve online. For example, users imagine they can purchase genuine, government-monitored prescription medicines without a prescription, or they are convinced by well-produced trademarks. On discussion platforms, users share their experiences with the medicines they purchased and advise each other to check for certain characteristics (such as a red stripe on the Kamagra package) in order to confirm the genuineness of the medicines. Consider, for example, the following snippet from an online discussion post:

> Yesterday I took my first BSB pill, wow it works fabulous. I had a dry mouth and did not sleep very well, but for the rest no serious side effects. I am taking a pill every other day, as I assume it is better for your body. Otherwise you might get used to it. So this morning I did not take another one, but I am still not hungry. I have to force myself to eat, I lost 1.7 kg in 2 days already.

It is worth noting how in online platforms medical information provided by other participants is often taken for granted, which makes users of these platforms easily prone to error (Attaran et al. 2011; UNICRI 2012; IRACM 2013). In addition, as outlined earlier, several studies have shown that online pharmacies do not list the risks of taking certain medicines, and that limited or inaccurate information was provided (Bessell et al. 2003; Wassink et al. 2010). Hence, as a matter of public health policy, these types of deceived consumers should be better warned of the health risks that may accompany online purchases.

On the contrary, *non-deceived consumers* are aware they are not purchasing medical products through legitimate sources and accept and take into account some form of risk. As one consumer of weight loss medicines highlights:

> It doesn't say anything on the ingredients list, but I think it will contain at least some kind of active ingredients. Otherwise it wouldn't work. I don't know what it is, I just think it is worth it as it helps me. . . . I know that it comes from China. I don't actually know where, but the language on the package is in Chinese as well. But it works for me, so it is ok I guess. Why would they suddenly sell bad medication?
>
> (Interview NC8)

Generally, neither deceived nor non-deceived consumers have a reliable technique or expertise for evaluating the quality, safety, and efficacy of products sold on the illicit market (Decorte 2001; Evans-Brown et al. 2009). In online markets, a 'quality check' is usually based on asking a friend who has ordered via the same website, 'trial and error' practices or reviews by unknown others, or discussing the online sources on forums and social media platforms (Van Hout 2014; Van de Ven 2016). Interestingly, for the non-deceived recreational consumers, quality in this context often refers to aspects such as reliability, purity, potency, and predictability of effect (similarly to what happens with illegal recreational drugs such as cocaine and ecstasy) (Bancroft and Reid 2015). Strategies to manage the risks of prescription medicines (primarily painkillers and opioids) in a socio-recreational setting are also often similar to the strategies employed to determine the quality of illegal drugs, alcohol, or hallucinogens (Quintero 2009). For instance, consumers' multiple tactics to determine the quality of the medicines might yield a wide range of beliefs regarding a medicine's quality. As one recreational consumer of various illicit lifestyle medicines responded:

> I received some sort of Ritalin and Viagra from a friend, but after two times I did not want to ask my friend for more. Some time ago I read some news on the Global Drug Survey and one of the conclusions was that if you purchase drugs online it is even cheaper and of better quality. So I think chances are quite high that the quality is good.
>
> (Interview NC9)

Similarly, consumers of sexual enhancers often reported their strategies to evaluate the quality while comparing it to the quality assessment of other illegal drugs. Yet, what makes the market for illicit medicines different from the quality checks in illicit drug markets is the fact that medicines can be purchased either legitimately or illegitimately. In his research, Quintero found that nonmedical consumers of medicines had a higher degree of trust in the consumption of medical painkillers than consumers of illicit drugs, because of the belief that prescription drugs are known and safe substances and because of personal knowledge (Quintero 2009:5). In this way, a form of medical trust seems to develop from consumers' own (positive) personal experiences, which, in turn, increases their confidence in other sources evaluating the quality and effects of pharmaceuticals. This was exemplified by respondents who claimed that they themselves would easily detect medicines of low quality.

Despite the similarities, consumers of illicit lifestyle medicines or human enhancement drugs do not perceive themselves as 'drug users' (McVeigh et al. 2012). Unlike users of illicit drugs like cocaine, consumers of medicines and other drugs for enhancement purposes often believe that the products they consume are fundamentally not harmful (McVeigh et al. 2012). This assumption leads them to apply less stringent risk management strategies, take higher risks, or sidestep risk management entirely because they are unaware of some of the potential risks.

Various scholars, including Monaghan (2001), argue that the use of certain human enhancement drugs such as steroids can be seen as a 'risky' lifestyle: for instance, bodybuilders who inject steroids in order to obtain more body mass take the riskiness of this (un)healthy behaviour and possible side effects for granted. In this sense, bodybuilding is an example of an ostensibly health-promoting lifestyle, even as report after report reinforces the message that steroid use induces health-damaging effects. These diverging health practices have been found also in my research, where it is very evident how many consumers of illicit lifestyle medicines are actively searching for medicines or specific ingredients that are not legally available, as they believe they are effective—no matter the risks. Consider, for instance, the experience reported by a Dutch health officer who wanted to inform consumers about the health risks of consuming online medicines:

> Recently we had cases of weight loss medicines that were sold online, but contained very dangerous ingredients, really very severe. So we posted a message on our website with the warning about the content: please do not buy these medicines because they are harmful. During a later study, we saw several forum posts where people were asking where they could buy these hazardous weight loss drugs. Because apparently the substance is very effective. But that was obviously not the intention of our message, we were aiming to warn people, not give them ideas to purchase illegal medication. (Interview NR10)

This quote highlights the risks consumers are prepared to take in an environment where enhancing their body's attributes appearance has become more important than having a healthy body (Nettleton 2013). While these risk-taking behaviours have already been acknowledged for hedonistic purposes, they have not been equally considered for enhancing purposes (see also Evans-Brown et al. 2012; McVeigh et al. 2012). Featherstone (2010) argued that in a consumer culture focused on adventure, pleasure, and living beyond conventions, the use of dangerous substances on the promise of attaining perfection (however this is understood by the consumer) are promoted. For this reason, body appearance may be even more important to the consumer than the body's health, as people choose to engage in potentially risky surgeries or use hazardous medicines or food supplements (Kraska et al. 2010; Nettleton 2013). Hence, it is important to understand more about consumer motivations and their risk management strategies also to better craft effective health-promoting messages: messages that focus on the availability of dangerous but effective substances not only fail to prevent people from purchasing these medicines online but may also actively stimulate others to look for medications that can enhance their beauty or wellbeing (whilst often being detrimental to their health).

To sum up, grounded on the existing literature and research data, a continuum of risk perception can be identified among consumers of online medical products: on the one extreme we find consumers who are prone to risks and are unwittingly consuming medicines as deceived consumers; on the other extreme, we find the non-deceived consumers who deliberately take risks into consideration for the wanted, often nonmedical, results (such as effective but harmful slimming pills). In the middle, we find consumers who take illicit drugs either for legitimate medical reasons or recreationally while being at least partially aware of the associated risks.

Conclusion

In this chapter, first-hand perspectives of consumers of illicit lifestyle medicines are used to analyse their motives and risk management of purchasing medicines online. As such, different analytical groups of online consumers of illicit lifestyle medicines have been outlined. Whereas some consumers have medical motivations for the consumption of medicines, recreational consumers take them for enhancement, lifestyle, or beauty purposes. Some buyers can be deceived into buying illicit products by, for example, illegal or fake online pharmacies, while other buyers are fully aware that they are purchasing medicines on the illicit market. It is therefore important to distinguish between medical and nonmedical consumers, as well as between deceived and non-deceived consumers of illicit medicines.

Consumers do not only differ because of their motivations for purchasing potentially dangerous substances online; as this study shows, they also differ in relation to the assumptions they have on, and management strategies they adopt to deal with, health-related risks. Generally (and similarly to users of medical treatments and therapies that are offered outside science-based medicine), online purchasers of illicit medicines have no guarantee of the quality of the medicines they purchase. Yet, based on this study it appears that, overall, users tend to have high trust in the websites they employ for purchasing illicit medication. While some users recognise the potential harms of these activities (at least to a certain extent), others seem to be more reckless and prepared to face serious health risks in their search for effective—even if potentially harmful—medicines. As consumers differ widely in their assumption and management of health-related risks, it is important for health care policies and policy makers to take these diverse motives and risk perceptions into consideration, and then target the different consumer groups with distinct health messages. Obviously, it is important to inform deceived consumers on the potential health risks associated with the purchase of medicines online. However, it should also be acknowledged that health messages will not always prevent non-deceived users from purchasing medicines online, and may even stimulate some to look for effective but harmful medications.

The results of this study suggest that it is therefore important to better investigate and understand the motivations (in line with Lavorgna and Di Ronco 2017), risk perceptions, and risk management strategies of people searching for health-related information online. Furthering this type of research is urgently needed in order to better design and target more effective interventions to mitigate the spread of potentially harmful information, products, and services online.

Acknowledgements

This chapter is based on the author's PhD study (Koenraadt 2018). This research project was funded by the European Union's Education Audio-visual and Cultural Executive Agency's Erasmus Mundus Fellowship.

The author would like to thank the editors for their helpful and constructive comments on this chapter.

References

Apodaca TR and Moser NC (2011) The use and abuse of prescription medication to facilitate or enhance sexual behavior among adolescents. *Clinical Pharmacology & Therapeutics* 89:22–24

Attaran A, Bate R and Kendall M (2011) Why and how to make an international crime of medicine counterfeiting. *Journal of International Criminal Justice* 9(2):325–354

Bancroft A and Reid PS (2015) Concepts of illicit drug quality among darknet market users: purity, embodied experience, craft and chemical knowledge. *The International Journal on Drug Policy*. Available at: http://doi.org/10.1016/j.drugpo.2015.11.008

Bechara A, Casabé A, De Bonis W, Helien A and Bertolino MV (2010) Recreational use of phosphodiesterase type 5 inhibitors by healthy young men. *The Journal of Sexual Medicine* 7(11):3736–3742

Benschop A, Nabben T and Korf DJ (2011) *Antenne Drugsgebruik 2010: trends in alcohol, tabak en drugs bij jonge Amsterdammers.* Amsterdam: Rozenberg Publishers

Bessell TL, Anderson JN, Silagy CA, Sansom LN and Hiller JE (2003) Surfing, self-medicating and safety: buying non-prescription and complementary medicines via the internet. *Quality and Safety in Health Care* 12(2):88–92

Blackstone EA, Fuhr JP and Pociask S (2014) The health and economic effects of counterfeit drugs. *American Health & Drug Benefits* 7(4):216–224

Brennan BP, Kanayama G and Pope Jr HG (2013) Performance-enhancing drugs on the web: a growing public-health issue. *The American Journal of Addictions* 2(2):158–161

Decorte T (2001) Drug users' perceptions of 'controlled' and 'uncontrolled' use. *International Journal of Drugs policy* 12(4):297–320

Di Giorgio D (ed.) (2011) *Counterfeit medicines: facts and practical advice.* Milan: EDQM-AIFA

Di Nicola A, Martini E and Baratto G (2015) *FAKECARE: developing expertise against the online trade of fake medicines by producing and disseminating knowledge, counterstrategies and tools across the EU.* eCrime Research Reports No.2, eCrime. Trento: University of Trento

Evans-Brown M, Kimergård A and McVeigh J (2009) Elephant in the room? The methodological implications for public health research of performance-enhancing drugs derived from the illicit market. *Drug Test Analysis* 1:323–326

Evans-Brown M, McVeigh J, Perkens C and Bellis MA (2012) *Human enhancement drugs: the emerging challenges to public health.* Available at: http://ldjjvvj.smmgp.org.uk/download/others/other076.pdf

Featherstone M (2010) Body, image and affect in consumer culture. *Body & Society* 16(1):193–221

Fernandez FM, Green MD and Newton PN (2008) Prevalence and detection of counterfeit pharmaceuticals: a mini review. *Industrial & Engineering Chemistry Research* 47(3):585–590

Gaudiono MC, Manna L, Rodomonte AL, Bartolomei M, Bertocchi P, Gallinella B, Antoniella E, Muleri N, Civitelli G, Alimonti S, Romanini L, Ruffini L and Valvo L (2012) A survey on illegal and counterfeit medicines for the treatment of erectile dysfunctions in Italy. *The journal of sexual medicine* 9(8):2130–2137

Gilbert D, Walley T and New B (2000) Lifestyle medicines. *BMJ: British Medical Journal* 321(7272):1341

Gott M and Hinchliff S (2003) Barriers to seeking treatment for sexual problems in primary care: a qualitative study with older people. *Family Practice* 20(6):690–695

Hall A and Antonopoulos GA (2016) *Fake meds online: the internet and the transnational market in illicit pharmaceuticals.* Basingstoke: Palgrave Macmillan

Hall MA, Dugan E, Zheng B and Mishra AK (2001) Trust in physicians and medical institutions: what is it, can it be measured, and does it matter? *Milbank Quarterly* 79(4):613–639

Heinonen JA, Spink J and Wilson JM (2014) When crime events defy classification: the case of product counterfeiting as white-collar crime. *Security Journal* 30(2):621–639

Intomart GfK (2009) *Geneesmiddelen op internet: een internet-onderzoek in opdracht van het ministerie van volksgezondheid.* Hilversum, NL: Intomart GfK bv

Intomart GfK (2012) *Risicogedrag bij het online bestellen van geneesmiddelen.* Hilversum, NL: Intomart GfK bv

IRACM (2013) *Counterfeit medicines and criminal organizations.* Paris: International Institute of Research Against Counterfeit Medicines

Ivanitskaya L, Brookins-Fisher J, O'Boyle I, Vibbert D, Erofeev D and Fulton L (2010) Dirt cheap and without prescription: how susceptible are young US consumers to purchasing drugs from rogue internet pharmacies? *Journal of medical Internet Research* 12(2):1–15

Jackson G, Arver S, Banks I and Stecher VJ (2010) Counterfeit phosphodiesterase type 5 inhibitors pose significant safety risks. *International Journal of Clinical Practice* 64(4):497–504

Koenraadt RM (2012) *Blauwe pillen op de zwarte markt: Een exploratief onderzoek naar het gebruik en de verkoop van illegale erectiemiddelen in Nederland.* Oisterwijk, NL: Wolf Legal Publishers

Koenraadt RM (2018) *In pursuit of a slim and sexual body: the illicit trade in lifestyle medicines.* Den Haag: Eleven Legal Publishers (diss. UU)

Koenraadt RM and de Haan M (2016) *De aankoop van geneesmiddelen via internet: Een onderzoek naar de aankoop, motieven en risicoperceptie bij het online bestellen van geneesmiddelen.* Utrecht: Willem Pompe Instituut voor Strafrechtswetenschappen

Koenraadt RM and Van de Ven K (2017) The internet and lifestyle drugs: an analysis of demographic characteristics, methods, and motives of online purchasers of illicit lifestyle drugs in the Netherlands. *Drugs: Education, Prevention and Policy* 25(4):345–355

Kraska PB, Bussard CR and Brent JJ (2010) Trafficking in bodily perfection: examining the late-modern steroid marketplace and its criminalisation. *Journal Quarterly* 27(2):159–185

Lavorgna A (2014) The online trade in counterfeit pharmaceuticals: new criminal opportunities, trends and challenges. *European Journal of Criminology* 12(2):226–241

Lavorgna A and Di Ronco A (2017) Fraud victims or unwary accomplices? An exploratory study of online communities supporting quack medicine. In Van Duyne PC, Harvey J, Antonopoulos GA and Von Lampe K (eds.) *The many faces of crime for profit and ways of tackling it.* Nijmegen, NL: Wolf Legal Publishers

Mazanov J, Dunn M, Connor J and Fielding ML (2013) Substance use to enhance academic performance among Australian university students. *Performance Enhancement and Health* 2:110–118

McVeigh J, Evans-Brown M and Bellis MA (2012) Human enhancement drugs and the pursuit of perfection. *Adicciones* 24(3):185–190

Monaghan L (2001) Looking good, feeling good: the embodied pleasures of vibrant physicality. *Sociology of Health & Illness* 23(3):330–356

Montoya ID and Jano E (2007) Online pharmacies, safety and regulatory considerations. *International Journal of Health Services* 37(2):279–289

Moreira ED, Brock G, Glasser DB, Nicolosi A, Laumann EO, Paik A, Wang T, Gingell C, GSSAB Investigators' Group (2005) Help-seeking behaviour for sexual problems: the global study of sexual attitudes and behaviors. *International journal of clinical practice* 59(1):6–16

Musacchio NS, Hartrich M and Garofalo R (2006) Erectile dysfunction and Viagra use: what's up with college-age males? *Journal of Adolescent Health* 39:452–454

Nettleton S (2013) *The sociology of health and illness.* Cambridge: Polity Press

Nettleton SJ and Hanlon G (2006) Pathways to the doctor in the information age: the role of ICTs in contemporary lay referral systems. In Webster A and Wyatt S (eds.) *Innovative health technologies: new perspectives, challenge and change.* London: Palgrave Macmillan

Nicolosi A, Buvat J, Glasser DB, Hartmann U, Laumann EO and Gingell C (2006) Sexual behaviour, sexual dysfunctions and related help seeking patterns in middle-aged and elderly Europeans: the global study of sexual attitudes and behaviors. *World Journal of Urology* 24(4):423–428

Orizio G and Gelatti U (2010) Public eHealth and new scenarios in terms of risks and opportunities: a specific focus on cyberpharmacies. *Social Semiotics* 20(1):29–41

Orizio G, Merla A, Schulz PJ and Gelatti U (2011) Quality of online pharmacies and websites selling prescription drugs: a systematic review. *Journal of Medical Internet Research* 13(3):e74

Paoli L and Donati A (2014) *The sports doping market: understanding supply and demand, and the challenges of their control*. New York: Springer

Peters RJ, Johnson RJ, Kelder S, Meshack AF and Jefferson T (2007) Beliefs and social norms about sildenafil citrate (Viagra) misuse and perceived consequences among Houstonian Teenage males. *American Journal of Men's Health* 1:208–212

Philaretou AG (2004) *The perils of masculinity: an analysis of male sexual anxiety, sexual addiction, and relational abuse*. Lanham, MD: University Press of America

Quintero G (2009) Rx for a party: a qualitative analysis of recreational pharmaceutical use in a collegiate setting. *Journal of American College Health* 58(1):64–72

Rahman SZ, Gupta V, Suhklecha A and Khunte Y (2010) Lifestyle drugs: concept and impact on society. *Indian Journal of Pharmaceutical Sciences* 72(4):409–413

UNICRI (2012) *Counterfeit medicines and organised crime*. Available at: www.unicri.it/topics/counterfeiting/medicines/report/Ctf_medicines_and_oc_advance_unedited2013.pdf

Van de Ven K (2016) *The formation and development of illicit performance and image enhancing drug markets: exploring supply and demand, and control policies in Belgium en the Netherlands* [unpublished Ph.D. dissertation]. University of Kent and Utrecht University

Van Hout MC (2014) SMART: an internet study of users' experiences of synthetic tanning. *Performance Enhancement & Health* 3(1):3–14

Venhuis BJ, Zwaagstra ME, van den Berg JDJ, van Riel AJHP, Wagenaar HWG, van Grootheest K, Barends DM and de Kaste D (2011) *Illicit erectile dysfunction products in the Netherlands: a decade of trends and a 2007–2010 product update*. Bilthoven, NL: RIVM

Venhuis BJ, Zwaagstra ME, van den Berg JDJ, Wagenaar HWG, Van Riel AJHP, Barends DM and De Kaste D (2009) *Trends in drug substances detected in illegal weight-loss medicines and dietary supplements. A 2002–2007 survey and health risk analysis*. Bilthoven, NL: RIVM

Wassink H, Coumans B and de Hon O (2010) *Gezondheidsrisico's illegale doping via internet*. Capelle aan den IJssel, NL: Dopingautoriteit

WHO (2012) *Substandard/spurious/falsely-labelled/falsified/counterfeit medical products: report of the working group of member states, sixty-fifth world health assembly*. Available at: http://apps.who.int/gb/ebwha/pdf_files/WHA65/A65_23-en.pdf

5 'First do no harm'

Exploring non-evidence-based practices within the Ukrainian health sector

Anna Markovska, Ganna Isayeva, and Sergyi Ostropolets

Introduction

Delivering effective healthcare requires safe, efficacious, and affordable treatments that comply with relevant international standards. To this end, effective interactions between government, policy makers, medical practitioners, and pharmaceutical sales representatives are important. In countries such as Ukraine, where the provision of medical services is underfunded and trust in medical practitioners low, the delivery of prescribed treatments through official conventional channels is poor, and patients tend to purchase drugs in licensed pharmacies without a prescription (Romaniuk and Semigina 2018). Consequently, the delivery of effective and safe healthcare may be compromised by systemic and individual forms of corruption.

Corruption has conventionally been defined as 'undue profit from the abuse of public authority' (Mungiu-Pippidi 2015:19). At the social level, corruption can be considered as 'an intrinsic part of a certain governance context, a social allocation mode' (Mungiu-Pippidi 2015:19). In the context of the healthcare sector, corruption can affect different phases of the value chain (Transparency International 2016)—from manufacture to distribution in the market—and take different forms, including the selling of pharmaceuticals prompted by the unethical behaviour of pharmaceutical companies and medical practitioners. The latter, in particular, can prescribe ineffective and harmful non-evidence-based over evidence-based treatments to their patients for personal gain (for instance, they can receive inducements from pharmaceutical companies).

Our working definition of 'non-evidence-based pharmaceuticals' includes drugs produced by otherwise legitimate pharmaceutical companies that have not been tested in accordance with appropriate international regulatory standards. In the social sciences, consideration of the use of non-evidence-based pharmaceuticals is relatively uncommon. To date, most studies have addressed this issue by focusing on drug counterfeiting, where unauthorised or fake versions of drugs are used as substitutes for genuine, approved products (Deisingh 2005; Davidson 2011). However, non-evidence-based treatments can also be used in other contexts, particularly in eastern and central Europe where the use of substandard pharmaceuticals generates unnecessary public expenditure and may harm the health of individual patients. According to the Anti-Corruption Centre (2018), 6% of drugs purchased in licensed Ukrainian pharmacies in 2017 were non-evidence-based. Moreover, four of the ten most popular medical drugs on sale in Ukraine lacked clinical approval for use in other countries.

It is worth noting that while many products described as 'prescription' or 'prescribed' in this chapter would require a script from a doctor to obtain them from a pharmacy in countries such as the United Kingdom; in Ukraine they are simply recommended by medical professionals and purchased directly from pharmacies without prescriptions. Balabanova (2012:1927) studied healthcare in post-Soviet countries and reported that Ukraine had the highest proportion of those who chose to self-treat 'despite stating that their condition was serious enough to justify seeking care'. Home-based treatment was regarded as being less expensive, with advice from pharmacies promoting it as being a substitute for accessing the costlier health system (Balabanova 2012).

We acknowledge that drug regulation is complex and often country-specific. While comparative studies in this area are limited, we aim in this chapter to develop a deeper understanding of the specific situation in Ukraine. Thus, this chapter contributes to the focused analysis of some systemic and individual vulnerabilities to corruption in the Ukrainian healthcare sector and the harmful social impact this type of corruption causes to the country. The first part of this chapter aims to critically address healthcare provisions and related corruption in Ukraine and analyse current trends in pharmaceutical sales at the national level to identify non-compliance with officially mandated medical standards through the prescription of non-evidence-based pharmaceuticals. Considering the nature and consequences of the high level of consumption of non-evidence-based drugs in Ukraine, the second part of the chapter presents the results of a small pilot study conducted at the National Therapy Institute (NTI) in Kharkiv that examined medical prescription patterns for cardiovascular patients.

Understanding systemic corruption in the context of the Ukrainian healthcare system

In the context of a widespread use of non-evidence-based drugs and home-based treatments that may cause serious harm to people, criminological research may prove to be especially enlightening. By focusing on the notion of 'social harm', often employed in critical criminology writings, it is possible to consider a full spectrum of criminal and non-criminal activities that can seriously harm patients (Hillyard and Tombs 2007)—including, of course, the selling and prescribing of non-evidence-based drugs. Greenfield and Paoli (2013) identified harm as a violation of legitimate interests of the key players and specified four types of harm and four types of bearers of harm. The four types of harm are functional (physical and psychological) harm, material harm, and reputational harm; and the four types of bearers of harm are individuals, private and governmental sectors, and the environment. More specifically, physical and psychological harm cover losses ranging from death to various degrees of pain and anxiety. Material harm covers a range of financial losses, while reputational harm concerns losses that arise from actions or events affecting others' view of the individual (Greenfield and Paoli 2013). In this chapter, corruption is discussed in relation to physical, material, and reputational harm. Pemberton (2007:36) notes that it is important to define 'the determining context that produces harms'. The government sector and state authorities are here contextualised as an environmental factor that enables opportunities for harmful practices.

After the collapse of the Soviet Union, Ukraine inherited a highly-centralised and oversized national health system, with on average 40% more hospitals and hospital beds *per capita* than in other EU countries (Fan 2015). However, following Ukraine's independence in 1991 and the country's subsequent economic downturn, this system remained largely unchanged with only limited reforms to address decentralisation (Lekhan et al. 2015). In the 23 years following Ukrainian independence, there have been 18 Ministers of Health, with 10 of them resigning within one year. Each new minister justified the lack of reform as being due to the ineffectiveness of other members of the government, a lack of official cooperation, and the inability of the system to adapt to change. This long neglect had a number of serious consequences. For example, life expectancy in 2012 was only 66.2 years for men (compared to a European average of 73.1) and 76.2 years for women (compared to a European average of 80.3). Cardiovascular diseases accounted for more than 60% of total mortality in 2010, significantly contributing to high mortality rates in the general Ukrainian population (Lekhan et al. 2015). Communicable diseases such as HIV and TB remain a serious concern in the country (Lekhan et al. 2015). In the last 10 years immunisation rates have fallen, leading to a significant increase in vaccine-preventable diseases (Lekhan et al. 2015); this is at least partially attributable to a lack of control over the quality of purchased vaccines. As a consequence of this inefficient healthcare system, public trust in medical practitioners is as low as is trust in state officials or representatives of the criminal justice system (Bekeshkina 2015).

Two principle features inherited from the old Soviet system were free healthcare provision and an absence of the economic evaluation of treatment outcomes. Article 49 of the Ukrainian Constitution (adopted in 1996) guarantees the right of all Ukrainians to receive free medical help in all state medical establishments (Verkhovna Rada 1996). In line with this approach, in 2002 the then Ukrainian government approved the *Directive for Providing the Citizens of Ukraine with Free Health Care Guaranteed by the State* (Cabinet of Ministers Resolution No. 955 of 11 July 2002). This provision consisted of a detailed list of healthcare services to be provided by publicly owned healthcare facilities free of charge and prescribed a standard of care (Lekhan et al. 2015; Romaniuk and Semigina 2018). For the first time, this directive introduced an element of state accountability in relation to an allocated healthcare budget, and standards were calculated according to predicted public access to medical practitioners (Lekhan et al. 2015). However, realistic costings for providing care free of charge according to these norms were not determined (Lekhan et al. 2015). This situation prompted healthcare providers to request semi-legal payments from patients and institutions, even though from a legal point of view hospitals are not allowed to charge for services. For example, in our study we found that most hospitals in the city of Kharkiv collect voluntary contributions at the point of hospitalisation on behalf of a charitable foundation (Mecenat).

In an attempt to address this situation, in June 2017 the Ukrainian Parliament considered adopting two decrees. The first (No. 6327) maintained the principle of free state medical assistance and was passed by Parliament. The second (No. 6329), which aimed at introducing state tariffs for medical help, was not passed, although it encouraged the approval of the first (Verkhovna Rada of Ukraine 2017a, b). Mrs Suprun, the then Minister of Health, stated that it is important 'to stop lying about the provision of free medical help for all, the truth is that the state cannot afford it' (as reported in *Segodnya* 2017). Mrs Suprun further remarked,

> MPs propose to leave all budgetary allocation for health under the control of corrupt state officials, though many disagree with the introduction of charges for citizens, because 'we have free medical help!' Do you see this free medical help? I only see the expensive cars of hospital managers whose official salary is ₴, UAH 6000 [£200][1] per month'.
>
> (*Segodnya* 2017)

This quasi-legal system of financing the health sector, therefore, remains tacitly encouraged by the state, which turns a 'blind eye' to unofficial payments made to medical staff (*Segodnya* 2017).

This practice of demanding so-called charitable donations is still widely practised with unofficial payments often required to receive urgent medical attention and medication (Lekhan et al. 2015; *Segodnya* 2017). We argue that the continued existence of a semi-legal payment system within Ukrainian health-care provision creates a challenging legal environment for all those involved. It maintains a situation where the Ministry of Health effectively operates outside legally defined norms and regulations and is thus unable, or unwilling, to enforce compliance with accepted medical standards. This consideration is important in the context of Greenfield and Paoli's (2013) discussion of harm as previously described: the general public perceives the actions of its government as being unprofessional, and the reputation of the authorities suffers as a result.

In 2015 the World Bank identified significant short-term priorities for the Ukrainian health sector (World Bank 2015). These were the provision of free medical care to all people in urgent need; a move to patient-based financing models; the reduction of waste; and the consolidation of facilities. Last but not least, the World Bank highlighted the need for increased transparency and accountability within the sector (World Bank 2015). Although anti-corruption initiatives have been introduced by successive Ukrainian governments, implementation was hindered by poor resource allocation, underinvestment, and rampant corruption in the sector (Fan 2015).

In 2014, for instance, the Ukrainian Parliament voted for a legislative measure to allow state procurement of prescription drugs to be temporarily (until 2020) delegated to a number of international organisations ('the 2015 anti-corruption reform', which we will encounter again later in this chapter) (Colborne 2017). Among the organisations selected were UNICEF, UNDP, Crown Agents (UK), IDA Foundation (The Netherlands), Partnership for Supply Chain Management, and Global Drug Facility (Switzerland) (Verkhovna Rada of Ukraine 2017). In 2016 this new system reduced the expenditure of the Ministry of Health of Ukraine by about £30m (*Daily* 2017). As an example of how this was achieved, consider that Crown Agents (UK) was given the task of supplying drugs for cancer patients and ended up paying 45% less than the Ukrainian Ministry of Health for the same drugs. While this new procurement system has demonstrated to be effective in curbing costs, it had the unintended consequences of displacing corruption deeper into the system where it may be less apparent: corrupt practices have indeed reportedly moved from the major cities to remote regions where their emergence is more problematic (*Segodnya* 2017). For example, the advocacy group Patients of Ukraine (2018) reported that, despite success in tackling corrupt drug procurement at state level, they nevertheless observed an increase in corruption affecting procurement in medium- and small-size hospitals. Such displacement of corrupt practices is hardly surprising in systemically corrupt organisations and emphasises the importance of understanding regional compliance in Ukraine with established national and international standards. The further from the centre a hospital is, the less likely it is to be monitored effectively and thus more opportunity will exist for corrupt conduct.

Over the past 25 years, criminologists have studied the issue of corruption and state crime in Eastern Europe in terms of its 'eradication' and the 'restoration of a good equilibrium' (Mungiu-Pippidi 2015:11). These objectives were supported by foreign donors who financed anti-corruption projects, with the aim of developing a series of legislative tools to fight it (Mungiu-Pippidi 2015). As a result of several post 2014 anti-corruption initiatives, in 2018 the National Anti-Corruption Bureau (NABU) of Ukraine was able to report that more than 90% of cases of corruption within the social sphere were healthcare-related (NABU 2018). According to NABU (2018), the most commonly breached articles of the Criminal Code of Ukraine relating to healthcare were Article 191 regulating 'misappropriation, embezzlement or conversion of property by the abuse of official position' and Article 368 concerning the 'accepting of an offer, promise or improper advantage by an official occupying a responsible position'. Criminality in healthcare is generally opportunistic in nature and ranges from the mismanagement of budgetary funds in the procurement of vaccines (*Segodnya* 2011), to the over-prescription of tests and pharmaceuticals by medical practitioners (Patients of Ukraine 2017). At each level of the healthcare hierarchy, opportunities exist for healthcare professionals to abuse the system, largely because of the non-enforcement of existing rules and standards.

One approach to investigate financial harm and corruption within the health sector is to analyse trends in pharmaceutical sales in Ukraine by studying whether evidence-based criteria are used in the prescription of pharmaceuticals and analysing the cost of drugs borne by patients.

The pharmaceutical market in Ukraine and the potential for individual corruption

Ukraine has the largest pharmaceutical production capacity of any of the countries of the former Soviet Union (*Delo* 2016). In 2015, there were 620 licensed pharmaceutical manufacturers in the country. All these pharmaceutical manufacturing companies are privately owned. According to the most recent estimates, domestic producers account for 28.2% of pharmaceutical consumption by value but 71.8% by volume, given that most domestic production is of low-cost generics (Deloitte 2013). In 2013, out of the 10 leading pharmaceutical manufacturers supplying the Ukrainian market, four were domestic producers. According to the State Medicines Service, in that same year there were 15,831 licensed pharmacies in Ukraine. These retail pharmacies supplied 79% of all pharmaceuticals directly to the population, while the remaining 21% were dispensed through hospitals (Iberglobal 2016). Table 5.1 shows the top 25 pharmaceutical companies by sales in Ukraine.

Table 5.1 Top 25 pharmaceutical companies by sales in Ukraine (2014–2016) compiled based on the CAC (2018) analysis

Pharmaceutical company	*2016*	*2015*	*2014*
Farmak (Ukraine)	1	1	1
Arterium Corporation (Ukraine)	2	5	5
Darnica (Ukraine)	3	3	4
Teva (Israel)	4	4	3
Berlin-Chemie (Germany)	5	2	2
Sanofi (France)	6	7	7
Zdorovie Gruppa (Ukraine)	7	6	9
Takeda (Japan)	8	8	6
Kiev Vitamin Factory (Ukraine)	9	11	15
KRKA (Slovenia)	10	10	10
Sandoz (Switzerland)	11	12	11
Gedeon Richter (Hungary)	12	9	8
Yuria Farm (Ukraine)	13	13	17
Kusum Farm (India/Ukraine)	14	14	20
Borshagovskiy (Ukraine)	15	15	18
Stada (Germany)	16	20	21
GlaxoSmithKline (UK)	17	16	16
Servier (France)	18	18	12

Pharmaceutical company	*2016*	*2015*	*2014*
Bayer Consumer Care (Switzerland)	19	17	14
Acino-Pharma Start (Ukraine)	20	23	29
Abbott Products GmbH (Germany)	21	21	19
Sopharma (Bulgaria)	22	22	27
Alpen Pharma AG (Switzerland)	23	25	22
Delta Medikel (Ukraine)	24	26	23
GlaxoSmithKline Consumer Healthcare (UK)	25	19	13

An analysis of the sales of the pharmaceutical companies presented in Table 5.1 demonstrates that sales of more expensive drugs by international companies (such as Sanofi) can outrank those of less expensive Ukrainian produced generics. For example, Plavix is produced by Sanofi (sixth on the table) and can be purchased from pharmacies for £37 per box, while generics can be produced by Ukrainian companies and purchased for only £2–4 per box. Practitioners who prescribe Plavix produced by Sanofi would be aware of the availability of cheaper generic drugs with the same active ingredient. This may be an indication that doctors may be incentivised by Sanofi to prescribe their products. In 2016, data suggests that the 'best-selling' drugs were not evidence-based. Top of the ranking was Actovegin (by Takeda), followed by No-Spa (Drotaverine, by Sanofi). These drugs are marketed directly to consumers in Ukraine. It is also interesting to note that (imported) aspirin, which is an evidenced-based medication, is at 14th place, while locally produced and cheaper aspirin does not appear in the ranking at all (Apteka 2016).

The Anti-Corruption Centre (2018) study suggests that year sales of evidence-based medical drugs amounted to 69.9% of the total volume of drug sales through pharmacies in Ukraine. The remainder consisted of the following categories of non-evidence-based pharmaceuticals: 2.1% on homeopathy; 6.1% on plant-based medical drugs; 17.9% on non-evidence-based medical drugs (such as Actovegin, a deproteinized hemoderivative from the blood of calves); and 4.0% on drugs that are not included in medical protocols for treatment (such as Hidazepam, an atypical benzodiazepine derivate developed in the Soviet Union but not registered anywhere else in the world). The cost of these drugs (both evidence- and non-evidence-based) per pack varied dramatically. In 2017 the average price of drugs, which were not listed in modern medical protocols, was ₴, UAH 40.7 (£1.14); plant-based medical drugs cost on average ₴, UAH 41.4 (£1.18); evidence-based drugs cost ₴, UAH 65.7 (£1.88); and the price of homeopathic drugs amounted to ₴, UAH 186.2 (£5.33) (ACC, 2017). The non-evidence-based drugs are noticeably more expensive in this list. As a result, an average Ukrainian family spent ₴, UAH 350 (£10) per year on non-evidence-based treatments. The average wage determined by the government was around £125 per month in 2018, and the average monthly wage in the capital Kiev was reported as being £230 (Trading Economics 2018).

What this suggests is that in Ukraine, where there is a low level of trust in medical professionals, there is a correspondingly high level of consumption of non-evidence-based drugs. These drugs are often purchased at a cost that is higher than that of evidence-based drugs. This is significant in that recent studies suggest that Ukrainians often avoid seeking professional medical help due to the cost of those medications recommended or prescribed (ACC 2017; *Censor* 2017).

The question remains as to the extent to which the doctor (who prescribes a particular drug over another) might benefit financially from making such prescriptions. This question is closely related to the concept of 'reputational harm' that in context of our study relates to the medical practitioners (Greenfield and Paoli 2013). There are a number of practices that occur in Ukraine that appear to link pharmaceutical companies to individual doctors. Anecdotal evidence suggests that a so-called system of loyalty between patients and doctors is widespread but has not been well researched. One aspect of this is that in theory patients carry cards that are intended to provide them with drugs at a reduced price (Orange Card 2017). In practice, these cards may encourage doctors' non-evidence-based prescribing practices. Each card carries a number that is identified with the doctor who prescribes a patients' treatment. In the course of informal conversations with Ukrainian medical doctors during the summer of 2017, we learned that doctors receive these so-called loyalty cards from the representatives of pharmaceutical companies to issue to their patients. Representatives of the company visit doctors monthly to check on and discuss

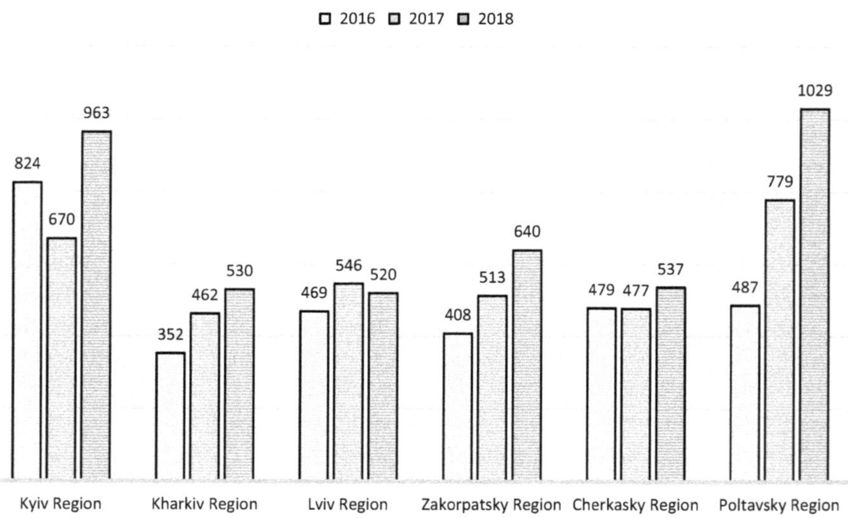

Figure 5.1 Spending on medical drugs based on the data provided by the Index of Health Ukraine (in ₴, UAH, from 2016 to 2018)

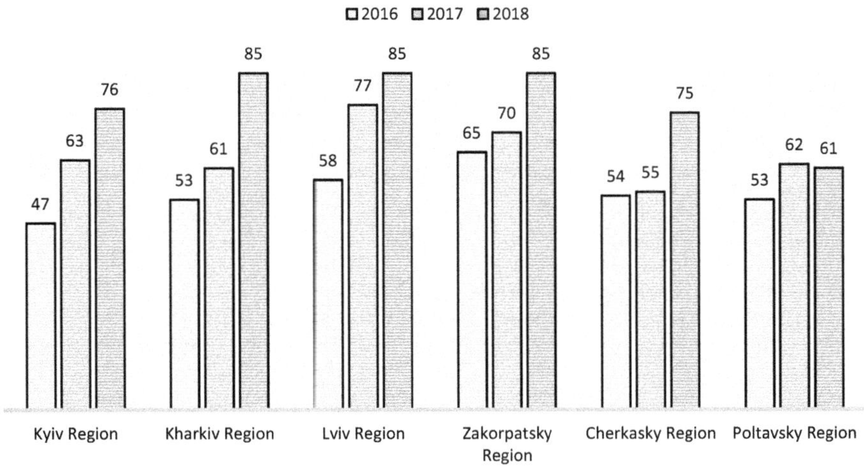

Figure 5.2 Number of patients avoiding medical attention due to the prohibitive cost of drugs

their prescribing practices. While this initiative may seem to reduce the cost of drugs to the patient (as on the presentation of this card at the pharmacy the patient is able to buy drugs at a reduced cost), its underlying motivation on the part of doctors and pharmaceutical companies remains questionable.

It is interesting to note that, according to the Programme Index of Health Ukraine, patients' spending on all medical drugs is rising across all regions, as shown in Figure 5.1.

The economic recession that followed the Maidan revolution devalued the Ukrainian currency, consequently increasing the proportion of the population living below the poverty line from 15% in 2014 to 25% in 2015 (World Bank 2015). At the same time, the pharmacy price of medical drugs increased. This resulted in a reported increase in the number of those patients who cannot afford to buy medical drugs and therefore avoid seeking medical attention (see Figure 5.2).

This trend deserves to be explored further as the Ukrainian population relies increasingly on self-treatment, and pharmacies have a significant influence on what medical drug patients will choose to purchase. The opportunities for pharmacies, medical practitioners, and the pharmaceutical companies that supply their medicaments to exploit patients are therefore extensive.

ACC (2017) reported on the top 10 most popular drugs Ukrainians purchased in pharmacies in 2017. Although the data is general and not classified according to disease, Actovegin is listed. Actovegin featured also in our cardiovascular disease pilot study in the list of non-evidence-based drugs frequently prescribed by doctors (see Table 5.2).

Four of the drugs in Table 5.2 (highlighted in bold) are non-evidence-based medicines. Understanding the complexities of the data and how it relates to the

Table 5.2 Top 10 medical drugs purchased in pharmacies in Ukraine

Medical drug	*2017 (₴, UAH in Millions)*
Nimesil (Nimesulide)	349
Actovegin	**342**
Sodium chloride	268
Nalbuphine	264
Xarelto (Rivaroxaban)	263
Spazmalgon (Metamizole Sodium)	244
Heptral (Ademetionine)	**225**
Seretide Diskus (Salmeterol+fluticasone)	217
Rheosorbilact (electrolytes+sorbitol)	**210**
Essentiale forte H (essential phospholipids)	**209**

realities of life in Ukraine is challenging. Although the consumption of non-evidence-based drugs in Ukraine has seen a slight decline, the consequences of people's reliance on the semi-legal health system discussed previously go beyond the issue of over-spending and indicate an increasing re-direction of patients from effective medical treatment to self-treatment, potentially creating socially harmful conditions. This type of harm can be considered, according to the classification of Greenfield and Paoli (2013), as physical and directly affecting the health and recovery of patients. Results from focus groups directed by the Patients of Ukraine Group (2017) suggest that one in two Ukrainians avoid seeking medical help due to the high cost of their medicines. For a majority of patients, the cost of medical drugs is prohibitive, and half of them are worried about counterfeit or low-quality drugs and the overprescribing practices of medical practitioners. Patients tend to be less aware, however, of the question of the prescription of non-evidence-based pharmaceuticals, suggesting that a public health information campaign would be a most useful way of helping the public to understand the issue.

Doctors' prescription practices in cardiovascular diseases: a case study

Prescribing practices are a difficult subject of study, one that is often avoided for a variety of reasons including the difficulty of accessing the required data without effective collaboration between medical professionals and social scientists. Our aim in this pilot case study is to explore the scale of non-evidence-based prescribing practices in 2014, and compare this with subsequent data from 2017, in order to assess doctors' prescribing practices in these two years (2014, 2017) also in the light of the 2015 anti-corruption intervention targeting corruption in pharmaceuticals' procurement, which may have reduced (together with other concurring factors) the prescribing of non-evidence-based drugs by doctors. We chose to focus on treatment of cardiovascular disorders, as these conditions contribute to about 60% of total deaths in Ukraine (Lekhan et al. 2015) and are highly standardised in terms of treatments as prescribed by the European guidelines (see the following paragraphs). We analysed data on prescribing practices at the National Therapy Institute in Kharkiv in November 2018; this is the first opportunity an independent researcher has had to analyse medical prescriptions in that institution.

The selection of case histories for analysis followed two stages. Firstly, the archive's administrator was requested to select case histories from 2014 and 2017; 236 cases were selected from 2017 and 251 cases from 2014. The administrator was then asked to select each fifth case registered in order to achieve the desired quantity of cases, which is 5% of the total number from both 2014 and 2017. Secondly, an independent researcher was employed to enter the data from these case histories into a spreadsheet. The resulting database included the following parameters from each case history: diagnosis, age of patient, oral prescription, and the duration of time spent in hospital. All patients selected had the same diagnosis of ischemic heart disease. Their prescribed drugs were analysed according to current European guidelines as represented by the ESC Scientific Document Group; ESC/EAS Guidelines for the Management of Dyslipidaemias; ESC Guidelines on diabetes, pre-diabetes, and cardiovascular diseases as developed in collaboration with the EASD; ESC/ESH Guidelines for the management of arterial hypertension; and ESC Chronic Coronary Disease (Montalescot et al. 2013; Rydén et al. 2013; Catapano et al. 2016; Williams et al. 2018).

The main characteristics of the patients are summarised in Table 5.3. The selected groups were broadly similar, and the results obtained between 2014 and 2017 were comparable. The analysis of these histories was conducted in the cardiovascular therapy department and excluded invasive treatments.

In our analysis, we first divided the medical drugs prescribed to patients according to the European evidence-based effectiveness indicators for the treatment of ischemic heart disease (Williams et al. 2018). The drugs that are recommended by the official European guidelines as having demonstrable efficacy are the following: aspirin, clopidogrel, angiotensin converting enzyme inhibitors, beta-adrenoreceptor blockers, diuretics, and ivabradine (Williams et al. 2018). Prescribed drugs that are not recommended by official guidelines for ischemic heart disease treatment and do not have an evidence-based background are

Table 5.3 Clinical characteristics of patients included in the sample

Characteristics	*2014* *n = 251*	*2017* *n = 236*	χ^2, *P*
Mean age, M±δ	58.3 ± 13.2	60.1 ± 11.4	0.109
Male/Female	171/80	143/93	3.01 0.083
Hypertension	209 (83.3%)	204 (86.4%)	0.95 0.330
Diabetes Mellitus	79 (31.4%)	71 (30.1%)	0.11 0.740
Heart Failure	204 (81.3%)	207 (87.7%)	3.85 0.050

quercetin, vinpocetine (Cavinton by Gedeon Richter), piracetam, L-lysine succinate, L-arginine, meldonium, armadyne, sulodexide, citicoline, carnivite (levocarnitine), Cerebrolysin (a peptide complex extracted from pig brain), and Berlition (bihioctic acid produced by the Menarini group). It is important to note that all the medical drugs assessed here as not clinically effective and non-evidence-based were prescribed and administered by injection, which is a more expensive way of administering drugs as well as a riskier procedure due to possible side effects (Hutin et al. 2003; Mallet et al. 2007; Panfilov et al. 2015).

Evidence-based medical drugs recommended for the treatment of ischemic heart disease were prescribed both in 2014 and 2017. For example, 248 (98.8%) patients were prescribed aspirin in 2014 and 229 (97%) in 2017. If aspirin was not recommended, the case history detailed the reason for this. Evidence-based Clopidogrel was prescribed in 2014 to 81 patients (32.7%) and in 2017 to 90 patients (38.1%). Ticagrelor was prescribed in 2014 to 2.7% of patients and to 6.3% of patients in 2017. The analysis of the data suggests that patients were receiving platelet aggregation inhibitors that significantly modified their prognosis. Statins were prescribed in most of the cases. In 2014, 249 (99.2%) and, in 2017, 213 (97.8%) of patients received statin therapy, a group of drugs that had a positive impact on treatment outcome. We further analysed data on the prescribing of beta-adrenoreceptors blockers and calcium channel antagonists.

Our results suggest that most patients in both 2014 and 2017 were treated according to the recommended guidelines, though in both years patients with ischemic heart disease were prescribed drugs of which the efficacy had not been demonstrated, most commonly quercitinum, meldonium dehydrate (Mildronate, Vasonate), vinpocetin (Cavinton), ethyl methyl hydroxypyridine succinate (Armadin), citicoline (Ceraxon, Neuroxon, Somaxon), propionate dehydrate (Metamax), heptral (Ademetionine), piracetam (Piracetam, Lucetam), and deproteinized hemoderivative of calf blood (Actovegin). We have calculated that for 208 patients receiving prescriptions for beta blockers made in 2017, 63 (30.3%) were also prescribed quercitinum. It is notable that in 36% of patients prescribed aspirin had also been prescribed quercitinum. Similarly, quercetin is co-prescribed for 30.8% of patients prescribed statins. It is important to note that the cost of 10 days aspirin therapy (dosage 100 mg Aspirin Bayer) is ₴, UAH 25 (£0.71), whereas the cost of 10 days treatment with quercitinum is ₴, UAH 1200 (£34.37). When we compare the prescriptions of statins and non-evidence-based drugs, we see similar data. The cost of a prescription of non-evidence Actovegin (400 mg per day) for 10 days is ₴, UAH 1300 (£37.23) and is regarded as being clinically ineffective. Our analysis suggests that treatment with non-evidence-based drugs requires patients to spend significantly more on their medication than they would do for only evidence-based medicines.

To sum up, in our study, most of the prescriptions issued in 2014 and 2017 were for evidence-based pharmaceuticals; however, a significant number of them were for (more costly) non-evidence-based pharmaceuticals. It is also clear that the practice of prescribing non-evidence-based drugs (see Figure 5.3) is not as evident in 2017 as it was in 2014, which suggests that the anti-corruption

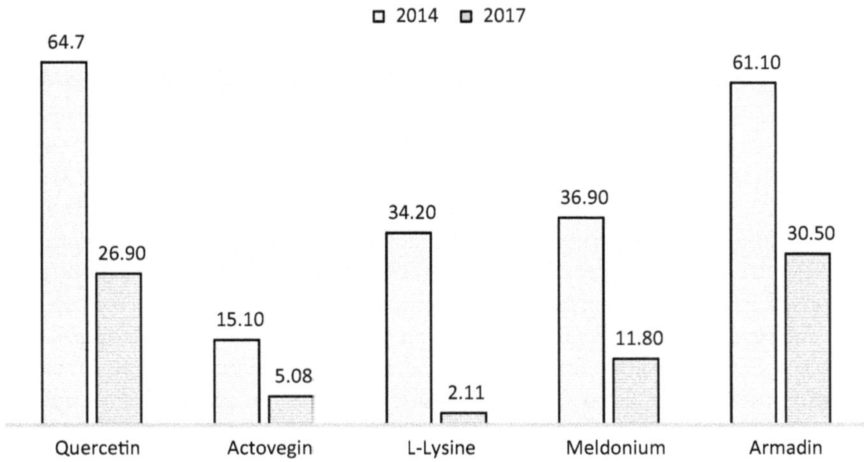

Figure 5.3 Non-evidence-based drug prescription dynamics 2014 and 2017 (no. of prescriptions per year)

interventions targeting corruption in pharmaceuticals' procurement may have had some positive effects.

Indeed, Figure 5.3 shows that 2017 saw a reduction in the prescription of all four selected non-evidence-based drugs in comparison with 2014. One possible explanation for this is the better enforcement of the standardised protocols that were established to comply with European guidelines (Ministry of Health Protection of Ukraine 2016). The practice of prescribing non-evidence-based drugs deviates from the standard protocols on treatment approved by the Ministry of Health. If these standards are not enforced, and the compliance mechanism is consequently non-existent, it seems clear that some doctors could be tempted to engage in dubious prescribing practices.

Conclusion

Systemic and individual corruption within the Ukrainian healthcare system leads to a wide range of harmful consequences. In particular, this chapter discussed the failure of the relevant authorities to improve doctors' compliance with official medical standards of treatment. As a consequence of this, a particular practice has been established whereby medical doctors over-prescribe non-evidence-based medical drugs. These prescriptions make some treatments too expensive for the general public. Questionable relationships between medical practitioners and pharmaceutical companies lead in their turn to the expansion of the socially harmful practices of self-prescription and self-treatment that are evident in contemporary Ukraine (ACC 2017; Gordonua 2017). In other words, corruption in the healthcare sector through the promotion of the prescription of non-evidence-based medicines can be responsible for both reputational harm to practitioners (and possibly for the medical profession as a whole) and physical harm to patients.

In the second part of the chapter, we presented the results of our pilot project studying prescriptions for cardiovascular patients. Our results suggest that 30% of drugs prescribed in 2017 were non-evidence-based. While most patients did receive evidence-based treatments (and, as such, medical standards were observed), recommendations and prescriptions for non-evidence-based drugs significantly increased the cost of treatment to the patient. The prescription of non-evidence-based pharmaceuticals suggests the existence of possible clandestine mechanisms of collusion, and potentially corrupt practices, between medical professionals and representatives of pharmaceutical companies. We suggest that the anti-corruption campaign initiated in 2014 to improve compliance with the European guidelines on medical treatment might (possibly in combination with other factors) have partially succeeded in reducing corrupting influences on doctors' prescription practices. In this pilot, we observed that the enforcement of medical standards and approved treatment regimes in the management of cardiovascular disorders might also have led to a decrease in the prescription of non-evidence-based therapies by 2017 as compared to 2014, although it has not eliminated the practice. We argue therefore that the enforcement of transparent standards is crucial to the suppression of the prescription of non-evidence-based drugs.

Note

1 1GBP=₴, UAH 34.9 (www.xe.com/currencyconverter), April 2019.

References

Anti-Corruption Centre (2018) *Pharmaceutical market in Ukraine*. Kiev: Renaissance Foundation

Apteka (2016) Sales of medical drugs in Ukraine in 2016. Available at: www.apteka.ua/article/388848

Balabanova D, Roberts B, Richardson E, Haerpfer C and McKee M (2012) Health care reform in the former Soviet Union: beyond the transition. *Health Services Research* 47(2):840–864

Bekeshkina I (2015) The significant decrease of trust in state officials. Available at: www.segodnya.ua/ukraine/doverie-ukraincev-k-vlastyam-rezko-uhudshilos-issledovanie-679356.html

Catapano AL, Graham I, De Backer G, Wiklund O, Chapman MJ, Drexel H, Hoes AW, Jennings CS, Landmesser U, Pedersen TR, Reiner Ž, Riccardi G, Taskinen MR, Tokgozoglu L, Verschuren WM, Vlachopoulos C, Wood DA, Zamorano JL and ESC Scientific Document Group (2016) ESC/EAS Guidelines for the management of dyslipidaemias/the task force for the management of dyslipidaemias of the European Society of Cardiology (ESC) and European Atherosclerosis Society (EAS). *European Heart Journal* 37(39):2999–3058

Censor (2017) 69% of Ukrainians are engaged in self-treatment due to lack of funds. Available at: https://censor.net.ua/news/458721/69_ukraintsev_zanimayutsya_samolecheniem_izza_nehvatki_sredstv_suprun

Colborne M (2017) Tackling pharma corruption in Ukraine. *CMAJ* 189(34):E1101–E1102

Daily (2017) Cheap but later than planned. Available at: www. daily.rbc.ua

Davidson M (2011) *Pharmaceutical anti-counterfeiting: combating the real danger from fake drugs*. London: Wiley

Deisingh AK (2005) Pharmaceutical counterfeiting. *The Analyst* 130(3):271–279

Delo (2016) Top ten most profitable drug manufacturers. Available at: https://delo.ua/business/top-10-samyh-dohocnyh-proizvoditelej-lekarstv-324515/

Deloitte (2013) Pharmaceutical industry in Ukraine. Available at: www.investin.if.ua/doc/pub/Ovewview_Pharmaceutical.pdf

Fan Q (2015) Ukraine's health system: time for change. Available at: www.worldbank.org/en/news/opinion/2015/04/06/ukraines-health-system-time-for-change

Gordonua (2017) Non-evidence-base drugs in Ukraine. Available at: https://gordonua.com/news/society/26-sredstv-kotorye-ukraincy-potratili-na-lekarstva-v-2017-godu-zaplacheny-za-preparaty-bez-dokazannoy-effektivnosti-issledovanie-326018.html

Greenfield VA and Paoli L (2013) A framework to assess the harms of crimes. *British Journal of Criminology* 53(5):864–885

Hillyard P and Tombs S (2007) From 'crime' to social harm? *Crime, Law and Social Change* 48(1):9–25

Hutin YJ, Hauri AM and Armstrong GL (2003) The use of injections in healthcare settings worldwide, 2000: literature review and regional estimates. *The BMJ* 8(327–7423):1075

Iberglobal (2016) Ukrainian pharmaceutical market. Available at: www.iberglobal.com/files/2016-2/ucrania_farmaceutico.pdf

Lekhan V, Rudiy V, Shevchenko M, Nitzan Kaluski D and Richardson E (2015) Ukraine: health system review. *Health System in Transition* 17(2). Available at: www.euro.who.int/__data/assets/pdf_file/0018/280701/UkraineHiT.pdf

Mallet L, Spinewine A and Huang A (2007) The challenge of managing drug interactions in elderly people. *Lancet* 14(370–9582) (Jul):185–191

Ministry of Health Protection of Ukraine (2016) On amendments to the order of the ministry of health of Ukraine dated Sept 28, 2012, No. 751 (12.29.2016 № 1422). Available at: https://zakon.rada.gov.ua/laws/show/z0530-17

Montalescot G, Sechtemn U, Achenbach S, Andreotti F, Arden C, Budaj A, Bugiardini R, Crea F, Cuisset T, Di Mario C, Ferreira JR, Gersh BJ, Gitt AK, Hulot JS, Marx N, Opie LH, Pfisterer M, Prescott E, Ruschitzka F, Sabate M, Senior R, Taggart DP, van der Wall E and Vrints C JM (2013) ESC scientific document group guidelines on the management of stable coronary artery disease the task force on the management of stable coronary artery disease of the European Society of Cardiology. *European Heart Journal* (34):2949–3003

Mungiu-Pippidi A (2015) *The quest for good governance: how societies develop control of corruption*. Cambridge: Cambridge University Press

OrangeCard (2017) Social programme 'orange card'. Available at: www.a.orangecard.com.ua/ru/

NABU (2018) The results of the national anti-corruption bureau of Ukraine activities. July-December 2018. Available at: https://nabu.gov.ua/en/report/report-second-half-2018

Panfilov SD and Panfilov DS (2015) Modern approaches to surgical treatment of post-injection vascular complications in intravenous drug addicts. *Angiol Sosud Khir* 21(3):134–139

Patients Ukraine (2017) Every other patient in Ukraine refuses from treatment because of high prices for medicines. Available at: http://patients.org.ua/2017/03/30/kozhen-drugyj-hvoryj-v-ukrayini-vidmovlyayetsya-vid-likuvannya-cherez-vysoki-tsiny-na-liky-rezultaty-doslidzhennya/

Patients of Ukraine (2018) Patients' organizations call Tymoshenko to stop manipulating the theme of international pharmaceutical procurement. Available at: http://patients.org.ua/en/2018/05/22/patsiyentski-organizatsiyi-zaklykaly-tymoshenko-ne-manipulyuvaty-temoyu-mizhnarodnyh-zakupivel/

Pemberton SA (2007) Social harm future(s): exploring the potential of the social harm approach. *Crime, Law and Social Change* 48(1-2):27–41

Romaniuk P and Semigina T (2018) Ukrainian health care system and its chances for successful transition from Soviet legacies. *Global Health* 14(1):116

Rydén L, Grant PJ, Anker SD, Berne C, Cosentino F, Danchin N, Deaton C, Escaned J, Hammes HP, Huikuri H, Marre M, Marx N, Mellbin L, Ostergren J, Patrono C, Seferovic P, Uva MS, Taskinen MR, Tendera M, Tuomilehto J, Valensi P and Zamorano JL (2013) ESC Guidelines on diabetes, pre-diabetes, and cardiovascular diseases developed in collaboration with the EASD. *European Heart Journal* 34:3035–3087

Segodnya (2011) The vaccine case. Available at: www.segodnya.ua/criminal/delo-o-vaktsinakh-arecty-i-ick-na-60-millionov.html

Segodnya (2017) Who will pay for our healthcare? Available at: www.segodnya.ua/life/health/reforma-zdravoohraneniya-kak-teper-budut-lechit-ukraincev-1028358.html

Trading Economic (2018) *Ukraine*. Available at: https://tradingeconomics.com/ukraine/minimum-wages

Transparency International (2016) Corruption in the pharmaceutical sector: diagnosing the challenges. Available at: www.transparency.org.uk/publications/corruption-in-the-pharmaceutical-sector/

Verkhovna Rada of Ukraine (1996) Constitution of Ukraine. Available at: https://zakon.rada.gov.ua/laws/show/254%D0%BA/96-%D0%B2%D1%80

Verkhovna Rada of Ukraine (2017a) Проект Закону про внесення змін до Бюджетного кодексу України [Draft Law on Amendments to the Budget Code of Ukraine]. Available at: http://w1.c1.rada.gov.ua/pls/zweb2/webproc4_1?pf3511=61568

Verkhovna Rada of Ukraine (2017b) Про державні фінансові гарантії медичного обслуговування населення. ЗАКОН УКРАЇНИ N 2168-VIII [On state financial guarantees of health services to population: law of Ukraine N2168-VIII]. Available at: https://zakon5.rada.gov.ua/laws/show/2168-19

Williams B, Mancia G, Spiering W, Rosei EA, Azizi M, Burnier M, Clement DL, Coca A, de Simone G, Dominiczak A, Kahan T, Mahfoud F, Redon J, Ruilope L, Zanchetti A, Kerins M, Kjeldsen SE, Kreutz R, Laurent S, Lip GYH, McManus R, Narkiewicz K, Ruschitzka F, Schmieder RE, Shlyakhto E, Tsioufis C, Aboyans V and Desormais I (2018) ESC scientific document group. 2018 ESC/ESH Guidelines for the management of arterial hypertension. *European Heart Journal* 39(33):3021–3104

World Bank (2015) Ukraine's health sector: time for change. Available at: www.worldbank.org/en/news/opinion/2015/04/06/ukraines-health-system-time-for-change

6 'Don't trust the experts!'

Analysing the use of populist rhetoric in the anti-vaxxers discourse in Italy

Ester Massa

Introduction

The healthcare system, its effectiveness, and the ways to improve it have become central and contested topics in the current political and social arena. At the core of this debate is the essential practice of immunisation. Recent data from the World Health Organization suggests a general lower level of vaccine confidence in the European region compared to other areas of the world (WHO 2018), and already in 2016 Larson had pointed out that seven of the ten countries with the lowest levels of safety-based confidence issues were European. This aspect is reflected in the actual data on vaccines' coverage, showing how between 2000 and 2017 routine child immunisation coverage of the first dose of measles-mumps-rubella (MMR) vaccine had decreased in nine EU member states, making the rate of confirmed measles cases in 2017 the highest since 2010 (WHO 2017). A similar trend can be found in the United States, where the percentage of non-immunised children has increased from 0.3% in 2001 to 1.3% for children born in 2015 (Hill et al. 2018).

Many reasons have triggered this rise in vaccine refusal, ranging from the specific political and social characteristics of the different countries to the varying attitudes of family GPs regarding vaccines (Larson et al. 2018). Not all these reasons can be addressed exhaustively in this contribution, which will only focus on the connections between the narrative proposed by populist movements and the way laypeople tend to address the issue of children's mandatory vaccinations. One very interesting remark in the previously mentioned report by Larson and colleagues has to do with the influence that anti-vaccine groups, aided by social and mainstream media, have had on spreading the wave of vaccine hesitancy, becoming somehow a factor able to impact on, and feedback into, political discourses on healthcare and immunisation practices. In this contribution, I will outline how this has also been made possible by the rise of a group of populist parties and movements especially during the first two decades of the new millennium, which have appropriated, nurtured, and diffused anti-vaccination arguments. They have done so by undermining the credibility of social and political elites and thus political and scientific experts, replacing the latter with new self-proclaimed 'experts' or 'expert elites'.

Distrust in the political system is nothing new; however, distrust in experts and scientists—those whose ideas, until the mid-20th century, represented the ultimate form of knowledge, whose opinion was trusted blindly (Giddens 1990)—is something quite recent. Collins and Evans (2008) called this phenomenon 'scientific populism'. Today, scientific populism applies to many common, tangible issues that affect the daily lives of millions of people, such as climate change or healthcare. In relation to issues so relevant to their lives, many people choose to disregard their highly technical nature and think they have a right to express a view, thus considering their opinions just as valid—if not even more valid!—as those of experts.

This contribution focuses specifically on the pro-vax vs anti-vax debate around children's mandatory vaccinations in Italy, a country where a populist government has used anti-vax arguments in order to generate consensus and consolidate its political power. A thematic analysis will compare the main themes emerging from the comments to an online newspaper article published on Facebook about an anti-vax rally held in Italy in 2019 (organised by anti-vaxxers to protest against a new immunisation regime introduced in 2017) and those emerging from the main rhetoric used by populist political representatives in dealing with the topic of children's immunisation (as retrieved from public interviews and newspaper articles). This chapter suggests that the distrust of experts heralded by populist parties and movements also supports and fuels the arguments used by laypeople to oppose official immunisation practices. It will be argued that the de-legitimising of experts is one the most troublesome traits of populist rhetoric, causing negative effects in society, especially in terms of decreasing immunisation levels and limiting popular awareness about fundamental facts about individual and general healthcare.

Political populism and the case of Italy

In order to understand the main themes that animate recent debates about healthcare, it is useful to briefly clarify what populism is and what its main contemporary features are. Scholars do not agree on a common definition of 'populism' (Rovira Kaltwasser 2015). For the purposes of this contribution, we will focus on the main element of interest within populist movements: that is, that of considering society as ultimately split into two homogeneous and antagonistic camps, 'the pure people'—i.e., the mainstream population who need to follow the rules—versus 'the corrupt elite'—those responsible for the production of the rules and society's status quo (Mudde 2004:543). Of course, the identification of these two opposing groups and their features may differ, demonstrating very different models of society and implying the inclusion or exclusion of very different social groups (Rovira Kaltwasser 2015).

Most of the new populist parties and political movements that have risen in the last few years belong to a nationalist, right-wing perspective (for instance UKIP in the United Kingdom, AfD in Germany, Front National—now renamed 'National Rally'—in France, and the Italian parties—The League and

Fratelli d'Italia [transl.: Brothers of Italy]). However, some of them have also been on the left wing (SYRIZA in Greece, Podemos in Spain), and at times (at least officially) have even rejected a binary distinction between right and left (like the Five Star Movement in Italy). Regardless of their political bent and official situation in the political spectrum, what all these movements share is a specific anti-establishment, rebellious stance and a declared distrust of previous political elites (that are thought of as detached from the people and not able to understand or represent their needs and requests). This is true not only for these (relatively) new and emerging political forces, but also for those movements that were already part of the political system, who over the past few years have tried to re-brand themselves to win back the consensus they once had. For instance, the change in the image of the US Republican Party (a mutation that has ultimately led to Donald Trump's election in 2016) is considered the product of a change in the meaning of the concept of 'class' in America, which has been defined by some as the 'great backlash' (Frank 2004): the working class (a difficult concept to define for many Americans) have ceased to be defined by their possessions or occupation and have started to be defined by personal characteristics, such as a certain unpretentiousness, humility, and attachment to solid all-American values (Frank 2004). In this successful re-branding of the Republican image, therefore, Democrats have been re-sketched as snobbish, over-educated people as opposed to the 'real Americans', effectively pointing at the Republican Party as the new 'working class party' (Nicholson and Segura 2012:371).

In Europe, the rise of populism has been sparked by the late 2000s' economic crisis, which has uncovered shortcomings in the design of European economic and political institutions (Acemoglu et al. 2013; Di Tella and Rotemberg 2016; Roberts 2016; Algan et al. 2017; Guiso et al. 2017). This started fuelling a distrust in traditional parties which led, on the one hand, to the rise of Eurosceptic populists—embracing the criticism of progressive values, such as cosmopolitanism and multiculturalism—and, on the other hand, to the rise of political extremism, which emphasises the culpability of the 'old' traditional moderate parties in causing contemporary economic insecurity (Algan et al. 2017).

Italy is a very good example of how the gradual distrust of European institutions, fuelled by the economic crisis, has led to the rise of populist movements, some of them totally new (the Five Star Movement) and others resulting from a successful re-branding of old political parties (such as Matteo Salvini's League, which successfully shifted its image from a territorially defined party advocating the independence of the northern regions from Rome's centralised power to a nationalist force willing to represent the Italian population against a perceived invasion of immigrants). Italians' traditionally favourable attitude to European integration has begun to slowly deteriorate since the 1990s, when also trust in the old political system started to crumble after some notorious corruption scandals (Roux and Verzichelli 2010; Serricchio 2012).

The progressive distrust towards the national and European political systems, however, has become increasingly evident especially over the last decade, fuelled by the austerity policies imposed by the 'stronger' EU members (such as Merkel's Germany) upon the 'weaker' ones such as Greece and Italy (Conti et al. 2016). In this climate of decreasing trust in the 'old' system and quest for the 'new' in politics, a window has opened for the entry of a new wave of political entrepreneurs onto the political scene, who have been able to interpret, and sometimes even re-direct, the main claims of many disillusioned people in Italy. The Five Star Movement, an internet party founded by a political TV commentator and comedian (Beppe Grillo) and a digital entrepreneur (Gianroberto Casaleggio), emerged as the most voted party in Italy in 2013 (with slightly over 25% of votes) (Ceccarini and Bordignon 2013; Conti and Memoli 2014). The Movement soon gained the support and allegiance of other parties, including the re-born Northern League under the leadership of Matteo Salvini (now simply called League), and the right-wing party Brothers of Italy. These anti-establishment parties and movements shared the same negative attitudes towards elites in general, who are perceived as guilty of granting favours to foreign powers to the detriment of Italian citizens (Conti et al. 2016). At the time of writing, the Italian government is led by a coalition made by the Five Star Movement and the League; the main populist traits that characterised their foundations are still very evident in all the main policies proposed and discussed until now—with the one about mandatory vaccines being one of the main battlefields in which the current populist war is being fought.

Political populism and childhood vaccinations: a hazardous relationship

Health issues are globally becoming more and more politicised, especially by populist movements and parties. Healthcare is, in fact, something that is very important to everyone, and public healthcare is something that involves and touches especially the weakest and more marginalised fringes of society (which are also the main targets for populist movements). The politicisation of health issues by populist parties encourages citizens to interpret the issue through a partisan perspective, leading to biased processing and motivated reasoning (Taber and Lodge 2006).

Many scholars have observed the interplay of politics in health and science communication (Nisbet and Huge 2006; Lupia 2013; Bolsen et al. 2014). Consider, for instance, the public response to the introduction of the HPV vaccine in 2006–2007 (Kahan 2013), or the uproar over the 2009 mammography screening guidelines in the USA—when the US Preventive Services Task Force lowered the recommended screenings (USPSTF 2009), thus sparking a major public debate on the balance between protecting women's health over saving government money (Franklin Fowler and Gollust 2015). The conflict lies mainly in the friction between the right of the state to dictate the direction of healthcare and the individual's right to be informed and have independence and governance over one's own body. One of the most polarising controversies, where the influence of populist movements is most evident, is the debate around mandatory vaccinations.

Although vaccination programmes are known to have eradicated or vastly reduced a number of dangerous diseases, preventing between 2 and 3 million deaths each year (WHO 2018), it has become clear in recent times that one of the worst problems in improving coverage, especially in European countries, is the so-called vaccine hesitancy—that is, parents' reluctance to vaccinate their children (Kennedy 2019). The origin of modern vaccine hesitancy is usually traced to an article in the renowned medical journal *The Lancet* in 1998, in which Andrew Wakefield suggested a cause–effect relationship between MMR vaccine and autism (see also chapters 3 and 9). The article has been since completely discredited, but nonetheless it produced an enormous impact on the general population, making the MMR vaccination rates in the United Kingdom, for instance, fall from 92% to 79% from 1995 to 2003 (Kennedy 2019). Ignorance and prejudice are usually used to justify vaccine hesitancy. Several studies, however, have recently suggested a different explanation, specifically connecting vaccine hesitancy to the diffusion of certain political views spread by populist movements.

As discussed in Kennedy (2019), the case of Italy, once again, is enlightening. The already cited Five Star Movement has in fact made one of the core points in its programme to raise doubts on the legitimacy and necessity of mandatory vaccinations. Beppe Grillo, the stand-up comedian inspirator and first founder of the movement, already in 1998 talked about these themes in a show (*Apocalisse Morbida*) that toured several cities in the whole nation.

> They cure you compulsorily, you are obliged to cure yourself. The principle is this: you take a healthy child and you inject in him a virus to get him used to it, and by doing so you lower his immune system. You inject into him a little tiny virus. In case the big virus came, the little virus is already there from years going through the body. But if the big virus doesn't come through, the little one is always there, it remains. And with the little virus there is also some mercury. We weaken our immune systems, we don't have any fucking defence anymore, we all have colds, cough, bronchitis, all the children need to stay in bed.
>
> (Grillo 1998)[1]

He also claimed, in the same show, that the contribution of vaccines and mandatory vaccinations to the improvement of the general health conditions in society had been grossly overestimated, since the incidence of some of the most dangerous diseases in the past had already started a downward trend before vaccines were introduced, and were naturally going to disappear:

> Diphtheria was naturally disappearing on its own, polio was disappearing on its own . . . In the Middle Ages you usually got ill, you died, nobody

> could see the bug because there was no microscope. It was God! At least it was God that made you fall ill, not a fucking multinational company!
>
> (Grillo 1998)

Since the ascension of the Five Star Movement in the political playground in 2013, the scepticism around vaccines has increased enormously, so much so that the MMR vaccination coverage in Italy has fallen from 90% in 2013 to 85% in 2016, resulting in an appalling increase in measles cases from 840 in 2016 to 5,000 in 2017 (John 2018).[2] It has to be clarified that, after exploiting their anti-vax proximity during the electoral campaign, after the 2018 Italian elections the Five Star Movement has somehow shifted its official position on mandatory vaccinations: many of the main leaders of the Movement now declare themselves not opposed to vaccines, but rather more in favour of a clearer information for the families, which can lead to some sort of informed choice, as opposed to obligations. This emphasis on information and on the individual right to decide, put in the hands of the parents, leaves room for some ambiguity, which certainly can still be exploited for gaining political consensus. The same ambiguity can be found in a recent event, dated January 2019, when, in a seemingly 'U-turn' fashion, Beppe Grillo decided to endorse the so-called Transversal Pact for Science,[3] an online appeal to all the Italian political forces promoted by two renown immunologists (Roberto Burioni and Guido Silvestri) with the intent of reaffirming the 'universal value of science for the progress of humanity'. A large part of the no-vax supporters of the movement immediately criticised this new position. However, considering what emerges from the words of the explicative post Grillo made on his personal blog (beppegrillo.it), the ideological change seems much less radical than it was thought to be:

> The ratio mathematics/reality still isn't completely clear. Science proceeds, without any fear through doubt (even coming to doubt itself). Science, and its world, need to survive, as anything else.
>
> (Grillo 2019)

It is certainly true that doubt represents one of the main driving forces in scientific research, but to justify this new position by highlighting this specific feature of scientific studies (and of scientists) somehow leaves a door open for the sceptics to maintain their positions intact.

In other European countries, similar situations can be found wherever populist parties have a say in Parliament. In France, the right-wing Front National raised concerns about vaccine safety and mandatory vaccinations; in Greece, the left-wing SYRIZA government tried to introduce the possibility for sceptical parents to opt their children out from compulsory vaccinations. In the United States, President Donald Trump gave a voice and support to the no-vax cause at the beginning of his mandate (Paun 2017). His official position changed very recently, though, after a severe measles outbreak, he decided to urge people to get vaccinations when directly asked by the White House reporters (*New York Times* 2019).

What further connects the inexorable spread in recent times of vaccine hesitancy to the growing consent around populist movements is the fact that 'scientific populism' (Collins and Evans 2008) seems to be driven by the same feelings of political populism—especially the distrust of elites and experts. The study run by Kennedy (2019) on the opinions of the people who voted in the 2014 elections for the European Parliament concluded that the higher the level of populist vote in a country, the greater the proportion of the population that believes that vaccines are not important or not effective. The correlation of the populist vote to the belief about the risk of vaccines has not proven significant, but nonetheless a close association between these two factors is evident. The anti-establishment narrative proper of the populist movements assigned personal agendas to scientific elites, essentially identifying their behaviours as that 'biopolitical control' over subjects or citizens that Michel Foucault (1976) had recognised—that is, the idea that control over people's health constitutes one effective way to retain power over the masses (Kaler 2009).

Methodology

The intent of the research presented in this chapter is to explore how the narrative mechanisms typically used by populist parties and movements relate to the ways laypeople tend to frame vaccines, and their refusal in particular. Officially, no government in the western world has adopted a clear anti-vax policy, but there have been some politicians encouraging a less strict obligation for children's compulsory vaccinations in several countries, including Italy. Here, a roaring debate is ongoing between pro- and anti-vaxxers also on social media (see also Chapter 9 of this volume). Consequently, the methodological approach chosen has been that of analysing the lot of online comments found on the Facebook page of the very popular Italian newspaper *La Repubblica*—a daily newspaper with a milder centre-left stance, and among the most-read newspapers in the country (ADS 2019), usually collecting comments from very different political sides—to an article contributing, somewhat neutrally, to the pro-vax/no-vax debate. Multiple voices have been found in the comments, making it possible to observe some of the key narratives used by people to support or oppose childhood vaccination; for the purpose of this study, only the main arguments used by anti-vaxxers in their discussions have been considered and analysed.

The selected newspaper article (Cravero 2019) focuses on a no-vax rally that was held in Turin, Italy, in late March 2019. The demonstrators' group, led by a spontaneous committee of concerned parents self-named 'Free to Choose', were protesting against the decision of the Italian Health Ministry to forbid the enrolment into schools of children who did not complete the whole set of 10 compulsory vaccinations. Originally down to a number of four, the mandatory vaccinations had been raised to 10 in 2017 by the previous government (law decree No 73 of 2017, the so-called Lorenzin Decree), unleashing protests from anti-vaxxers all over the country (see also Chapter 9 for a more detailed overview of recent changes in Italian vaccination policies). While several protests had been staged during the last couple of years, voices against mandatory vaccinations became more and more insistent after the last general elections upheld the new governmental coalition between the Five Star Movement and Salvini's League.

The article did not take sides on the matter, only reporting a neutral account of the rally and of the main examples highlighted by the protesters. However, the online commentators decided to ignore the article per se and to expand the conversation onto the main points of the broader debate on childhood vaccinations. The total number of comments up to the date of the analysis (15 May 2019) were 4,422, of which the vast majority were in support of the contested law and of the mandatory vaccinations. However, 87 commentators proposed strong alternative arguments in opposition to this new law, allowing the author to identify them as 'anti-vax commentators'. The comments clearly in opposition to mandatory vaccinations for children were approximately 323, representing the 7.3% of the total number of the comments to the article—a figure that gets pretty close to the latest estimate for the part of the population opposing mandatory vaccinations (8% in 2017) (Osservatorio Scienza, Tecnologia e Società 2017). These no-vaxxers' comments and the logic sustaining their main arguments have been the main focus of this study.

The methodology chosen for this contribution entailed a passive online ethnography (Murthy 2008) with observation of all the comments present in the website at the mentioned date. The manually collected comments have been thematically analysed to identify the most represented themes in anti-vaxxers' arguments. These themes have then been compared to those emerging from the selected publicly available interviews and speeches of the main political leaders of populist movements in Italy and in the United States. The exploratory study proposed here does not represent an exhaustive response to the question of the links between populism and vaccine hesitancy. It is limited to a very specific country (Italy), and it focuses on the analysis of comments to only one newspaper article posted by the newspaper outlet itself (*La Repubblica*) on Facebook. The latter is a very well-known social network, which nonetheless underrepresents certain sectors of the population. In addition, even those people regularly accessing the internet and having a Facebook account needed to follow *La Repubblica*'s Facebook page (which at the moment of writing, in May 2019, is followed by over 3,600,000 Facebook users) to have a chance of reading the article and leaving a comment. Of course, in order to have a better understanding of the main features and motivations behind the anti-vax movement, a larger sample of comments needs to be selected and analysed, possibly involving the observation of different social media and media in general (both print and broadcasted), in order avoid the risk of limiting the analysis to specific kinds of readers (e.g., with similar demographics and political views). A comparison with the opposed comments of pro-vax supporters could also add interesting reflections to the analysis. Nonetheless, this exploratory study only focuses on the main themes emerging from the no-vax side of the debate, contextualising them in the larger political and social climate in Italy and in the western world.

The ethical aspects of online research still constitute an uncertain ground for social scientists, with ethical standards being still under refinement. In line with the consensus that has been slowly developing in criminology and sociology on how to gather data online when those are created by online community users (Décary-Hétu and Aldridge 2015; Lavorgna 2015; Pink et al. 2016; Davies et al. 2017), this study has been conducted without a specific formal consent from the people who left comments under the selected article. Indeed, their voluntary submission of the comments on a Facebook page, having accepted and signed the site's privacy terms to enter the Facebook community, implies the public nature of the submitted comment. To protect users' anonymity, all the comments had been strictly anonymised in all phases of the research.

Results and discussion

Theme 1: 'We know better'

Based on a mix between self-made information, personal readings of highly technical information (including chemical and biological reports), and basic common sense, the anti-vaxxers' main claim is that of being more knowledgeable and informed about the actual composition, functioning, and, most importantly, risks associated with immunisation practices than the average person who decides to immunise their children. This emerges from the comments highlighting the incompetence of many of the pro-vax parents:

> They all 'have the blinkers', they don't see and don't want to listen. Maybe most of them don't even know which vaccines they children did. I asked to some young mums and they told me I don't know I need to see the vaccination book. And there are many of them.
>
> If only those in favour of the vaccines tried to investigate a bit more . . . they would never submit their children to such a practice.

Commentators do not only think that they are more informed than vaccinating parents; they also believe that they are more intelligent than them, because they are able to recognise the possible misdirection carried out by the authorities in order to maintain their power over people's decisions. The main evidence provided in support of these claims is the supposed 'authentic interpretation' of the description and therapeutic indication of vaccines as found in the inner leaflet present in vaccines' boxes. According to the anti-vaxxers' interpretation, there is a potential risk for those who undergo a vaccination to be infected with the disease they aim at preventing in the following six weeks from immunisation.

> Perhaps go and read the data from the OMS: in 2018 in Europe, the year with the highest vaccinal coverage, there has been a boom of infected people, included from the measles! This is because when you get a vaccine you are potentially contagious for 6 weeks! And the rush that is usually called 'little measles' is nothing but proper measles, and it is contagious! Those children, however, can go to pre-school or primary schools without any problem.

Another point made by anti-vaxxers is that infectious diseases have always existed, and yet in the past people survived them, receiving immunisation simply by being exposed to diseases and developing healthy antibodies. Consider, for instance the following snippets:

> My mother in the 70s with a box of mentholated balm worth 350 lire cured all of his children's rush illnesses.
>
> Prior to the Lorenzin Decree the mandatory vaccinations were 4. . . we are all still alive . . . we and our children had passes measles, rubella, mumps . . . the immunosuppressed can do them [the vaccines] . . . who didn't have the rush illnesses as a child can be immunised . . . but for the rest of the population I don't find the obligation fair . . . the freedom of choice in these cases is always the best thing.

When we look at the main rhetorical arguments in the speeches of political representatives for populist movements, often we find the same logic. In Italy, for instance, the Five Star Movement's elected representative Paola Taverna, who is currently the Italian Senate Vice President, infamously backed up the anti-vaxxers instances during a public debate claiming that, when she was young, 'when a cousin in my family had a sudden illness, we would queue to enter his house, so that my aunt could tend to all the ill cousins at once and all of them recovered from the disease for good' (*Corriere TV* 2018).

Theme 2: freedom of choice and self-determination

A second major theme in the vast amount of comments from the anti-vax supporters deals with the idea of self-determination and freedom of choice, especially in relation to health and wellbeing issues. Personal health is deemed more important than public health (preserved through the introduction of mandatory vaccinations, and especially through the achievement of a percentage of immunised people that allows the existence of the so-called herd immunity). Consider, for instance, the following snippets from the online comments analysed:

> For the immunosuppressed nothing changes if all around him are vaccinated. There are more than 100 illnesses without vaccines and many are very serious, I am not covered by any vaccine and I go where the fuck I want. You can fill yourself up with vaccines. My body, my choice.
>
> Maybe you should refresh your knowledge of the law and the constitution, last I checked children did not belong to the State!

According to anti-vaxxers' rhetoric, we should not be informed passively about health, but rather start to do our own research in order to make our own choices, without being conditioned by outer forces. The flaw, however, is right here: how do you get your information? Much of the anti-vax supporters suggest using the (perceived) unlimited freedom of information provided by the internet, inviting simply to 'google it'. It does not really matter if the information accessible is not usually verified, or that the results of this research can be easily biased. Consider, for instance, the following statement from the front page of the website Stop Mandatory Vaccination[4]—the reference website for one of the largest online communities of anti-vaxxers:

> When a parent who has a vaccine-injured child says to you, 'DO YOUR RESEARCH', that's why this website exists—so you can do YOUR research. Be brave, your children are counting on you!

The same logic, pivoting around the ideas of freedom of choice and self-determination, has been often used by politicians. One example is the recent legislative proposal by the regional section of the Five Star Movement of Lazio (the region around Rome), according to which we should overcome of the practice of 'coercive vaccination' to move towards 'personalised vaccination', and receive information on 'the causal link between vaccines and pathologies' and 'preventive nutrition' (Consiglio Regionale del Lazio 2018).[5] Similarly, consider the official statement given by the Health Ministry Giulia Grillo (another Five Star Movement representative) about the movement position regarding the Lorenzin Decree:

> The Lorenzin Decree, the one introducing the 10 mandatory vaccinations—just to be clear—is a law that we criticised already at the time of its approval. . . . We are in favour of the recommendation model, which acts on people's awareness and on the complete information about prevention. (Grillo 2019)

Also, Matteo Salvini (the leader of the League party) has repeatedly supported the argument of the need for comprehensive information in order to persuade families to immunise, as opposed to coercive vaccinations. He presents himself 'as a father who immunised his children, by choice and not because I was obliged, and knows the benefits, but also the risks, associated to this choice' and sustains that 'we must educate and accompany the parents, not oblige them' (Salvini in Lega Nord 2018). With this argument, while altogether affirming the importance of vaccines to preserve the general health in the country, he 'winks' at the anti-vax movement, essentially recognising the validity of certain doubts about vaccines' safety and necessity.

Theme 3: conspiracies and coverups

The third theme that is clearly identifiable in the anti-vaxxers comments to the selected newspaper article is related to the existence of a big pharma conspiracy (in line with Lavorgna and Di Ronco 2017). Experts are thought to be 'mercenaries' hired by big pharmaceutical companies with some sort of political agenda of their own. The same theme is often found when scientists' recommendations are attacked by populist leaders. A recent notorious example can be found in the debate about climate change, recently defined by Donald Trump as something akin to a hoax, because scientists 'have a very big political agenda' (Trump 2018). In Italy, the conspiracy argument is very evident in the public speeches of the already mentioned comedian Beppe Grillo. We already saw how the ghost of the big pharma industries has been pointed out as the reason for the mass vaccinations in his shows in the late 1990s.

The anti-vaxxers' websites and Facebook groups all over the world are filled with these conspiracy theories, and the Facebook page here analysed is no exception. Consider, for instance, the following examples:

> She has a closed mind, she doesn't inform herself she just makes reference to what she has been taught. A sheep in a sick social paddock. And pharmaceutical companies make money out of sheep!
>
> . . . I applaud who has been able to direct you. First of all medicine is NOT a science and you would understand it well if you were thinking as an individual and not as a mere piece in a herd.
>
> . . . The absolute ignorance that envelopes little people like you, daring to menace another human being just for asking truth and justice (which you cannot understand because you are blinded by an arrogant false knowledge of the vaccination issue) is a poison that is at the base of the poor condition in which humanity floats every day.

Another interesting perspective used as an argument to reinforce the idea of a political agenda of the authorities recommending vaccinations is the idea that authorities use vaccines to divert people's attention from more dangerous problems:

> Tetanus is not contagious.
>
> Taranto has a population of 200.000 people.
>
> Tetanus kills 0.05 inhabitants of Taranto each year.

> ILVA kills 1500 people each year.
>
> How comes that the State obliges the inhabitants of Taranto to protect themselves against tetanus and don't protect them from something that can kill them 30.000 times more?
>
> Is there a tetanus emergency or an ILVA emergency?

The illnesses the vaccines protect us from are considered as something somewhat rare in our modern world (like tetanus, in the example above); at the same time, other much more serious health problems, related to pollution and safety in the workplace, are ignored or not addressed with sufficient vigour (in the comment above, the example is related to the poisonous emissions of ILVA, a big steelwork factory in the Southern city of Taranto, which has been proved to be the cause of many illnesses and death by cancer over several decades).

A concluding thought

What seems fairly evident from this exploratory analysis is that each of the main arguments of anti-vaxxers (e.g., vaccines as unsafe; freedom of choice and right to self-determination in immunisation practices; the existence of a 'conspiracy' promoting mandatory vaccinations) could be easily challenged with the use of scientific evidence, usually reported to the public at large by trusted experts. It would not take long to reaffirm the validity of vaccinations if the informed opinion of immunologists and scientific researchers were heard and respected for their value. But here one of the mechanisms that informs the whole populist rhetoric comes into play: the complete distrust of authorities and traditional elites. Unfortunately, experts, even scientific ones, often come from the same elites, schools, or social classes that the current populist discourse blames for society's problems over anything else. Thus, to trust experts recommending vaccinations would be—in the view of those falling for populists' approaches—to listen to the same cultural base that produced the hated older generation of politicians, who are knowledgeable in political and business matters, but unfortunately too detached from the real population, and often corrupted.

This visceral disgust towards the former ruling class is a big part of the sentiment that gave way in Italy to the first 'Fuck you Day' in 2007 (a series of shows/rallies promoted by the founder and motivational leader of the Five Star Movement Beppe Grillo and designed to be a 'giant scream' against the 'official political regimes'), and that made people chant 'Make America Great Again' in Trump's electoral rallies during the last presidential elections. UKIP followers in Great Britain have supported politicians that claim to be closer to real people for years now, and the result of the Brexit referendum in 2016 can also be interpreted in the light of this will to get rid of traditional political elites.

Along this logic, professional politicians (with a derogatory meaning, as in bureaucratic, privileged figures, bred inside the traditional parties, far removed from the real needs of the people), scientists, and pharmaceutical entrepreneurs are mostly perceived as part of a 'caste' aimed at controlling the masses and pursuing personal power and economic interests. For this very reason, both sensible political arguments and scientific explanations should not be entirely trusted, preferring a more sceptical approach to vaccines based on personal research of the medicines' benefits and risks and of the possible interests at play. This resonates well with the basic ideals of direct democracy (at the foundation of many contemporary populist movements) but exposes the populations to the risk of great detriment to their own health and to society as a whole.

This exploratory study has shed some light on some of the populist movements' most common narrative mechanisms influencing the anti-vax debate in Italy. Future development of this line of research would need to explore more in depth, with a rigorous content (and even visual) analysis, how these narratives influence anti-vaxxers' arguments and frames on immunisation practices, especially with a view to identifying possible ways to increase confidence in scientific experts and reduce vaccine hesitancy.

Acknowledgements

I would like to thank Matt Clement for proofreading this chapter.

Notes

1 All the Italian quotes have been translated by the author.
2 However, more recent data present a relative increase in the measles vaccinations, making the national coverage at 94.3% as of 30th June 2018 (Ministero della Salute 2019), probably as a reaction to the public debate about the rise in the measles cases in the country in the previous years.
3 See www.pattoperlascienza.it/.
4 See www.stopmandatoryvaccination.com/.
5 See www.quotidianosanita.it/allegati/allegato9859338.pdf.

References

Acemoglu D, Egorov G and Sonin K (2013) A political theory of populism. *Quarterly Journal of Economics* 128(2):771–805

ADS (Accertamenti Diffusione Stampa) (2019) *Ultimi Dati Certificati (2017)*. Available at: www.adsnotizie.it/

Algan Y, Guriev S, Papaioannou E and Passari E (2017) The European trust crisis and the rise of populism. *Brookings Papers on Economic Activity* 2:309–400

Bolsen TJ, Druckman N and Lomax Cook F (2014) How frames can undermine support for scientific adaptations: politicization and the status-quo bias. *Public Opinion Quarterly* 78(1):1–26

Ceccarini L and Bordignon F (2013) Five Star and a cricket: Beppe Grillo shakes Italian politics. *South European Society and Politics* 18(4):427

Collins H and Evans R (2008) *Rethinking expertise*. Chicago: University of Chicago Press

Consiglio Regionale del Lazio (2018) *Proposta n.52 del 17 Luglio 2018*. Available at: www.quotidianosanita.it/allegati/allegato9859338.pdf

Conti N, Cotta M and Verzichelli L (2016) The economic crisis and its effects on the attitudes of Italian political elites towards the EU. *Historical Social Research/Historische Sozialforschung* 41(4/158):129–149

Conti N and Memoli V (2014) Italy. In Conti N (ed.) *Party attitudes toward the EU in the member states*. London: Routledge

Corriere TV (2018) Paola Taverna e i vaccini: 'Quando ero piccola per immunizzarci andavamo a trovare i cugini malati'. Aug 7. Available at: https://video.corriere.it/vaccini-ricetta-paola-taverna-a-casa-mia-zia-facevano-processione/a18e7eaa-9a72-11e8-b29e-fbb2c6c2bbaf

Cravero F (2019) Torino, oltre 1.500 No Vax in piazza: 'Basta esclusioni da scuola'. *La Repubblica*. Mar 23 Available at: https://torino.repubblica.it/cronaca/2019/03/23/news/torino_i_no_vax_tornano_in_piazza_no_all_obbligo_di_legge_-222308384/?fbclid=IwAR3Z9uv-qBhAHgJfnO5vaMcKCnLFWUyLmwFj1RFxJCJhybTLPOtDq29pwhI

Davies H, Halford S, Hine C, Hotz C, Martin W and Sugiura L (2017) *Ethics guidelines and collated resources for digital research*. British Sociological Association. Available at: www.britsoc.co.uk/media/24309/bsa_statement_of_ethical_practice_annexe.pdf

Décary-Hétu D and Aldridge J (2015) Sifting through the Net: monitoring of online offenders by researchers. *The European Review of Organised Crime* 2(2):122–141

Di Tella R and Rotemberg JJ (2016) *Populism and the return of the 'paranoid style': some evidence and a simple model of demand for incompetence as insurance against elite betrayal*. Working Paper No. 22975. Cambridge, MA: National Bureau of Economic Research

Foucault M (1979) [1976] *The history of sexuality volume 1: an introduction*. London: Allen Lane

Frank T (2004) *What's the matter with Kansas? How conservatives won the heart of America*. New York: Henry Holt and Company

Franklin Fowler E and Gollust SE (2015) The content and effect of politicized health controversies. *The Annals of the American Academy of Political and Social Science* 658:155–171

Giddens AT (1990) *The consequences of modernity*. Stanford: Stanford University Press

Grillo B (1998) *Apocalisse morbida*. Available at: www.youtube.com/watch?v=6HpcnoSgq0U

Grillo B (2019) Patto trasversale per la scienza. *Il Blog di Beppe Grillo*. Jan 10. Available at: www.beppegrillo.it/patto-trasversale-per-la-scienza/

Grillo G (2019) Sui vaccini non faremo passi indietro. *Il blog delle stele*. Mar 11. Available at: www.ilblogdellestelle.it/2019/03/sui-vaccini-non-faremo-passi-indietro.html

Guiso L, Herrera H, Morelli M and Sonno T (2017) Populism: demand and supply. Working Paper. Available at: www.heliosherrera.com/ populism.pdf

Hill HA, Elam-Evans LD, Yankey D, Singleton JA and Kang Y (2018) Vaccination coverage among children aged 19–35 months – United States, 2017. *Morbidity and Mortality Weekly Report* 67(40):1123–1128

John T (2018) *How anti-vaxxers could help decide Italy's election*. Available at: www.time.com/5165670/vaccine-skepticism-northern-league-five-star

Kahan DM (2013) A risky science communication environment for vaccines. *Science* 342(6154):53–54

Kaler A (2009) Health interventions and the persistence of rumour: the circulation of sterility stories in African public health campaigns. *Social Science & Medicine* 68:1711–1719

Kennedy J (2019) Populist politics and vaccine hesitancy in western Europe: an analysis of national-level data. *European Journal of Public Health* (online first)

Larson H (2016) The state of vaccine confidence 2016: global insights through a 67-country survey. *EBioMedicine*:295–301

Larson H, De Figueiredo A, Karafllakis E and Rawal M (2018), *State od vaccine confidence in the EU 2018*. Report for the European Commission. Available at: https://ec.europa.eu/health/sites/health/files/vaccination/docs/2018_vaccine_confidence_en.pdf

Lavorgna A (2015) The social organization of pet trafficking in cyberspace. *European Journal of Criminal Policy and Research* 21(3):353–370

Lavorgna A and Di Ronco A (2017) Fraud victims or unwary accomplices? An exploratory study of online communities supporting quack medicine. In van Duyne PC, Harvey J, Antonopoulos GA and von Lampe K (eds.) *The many faces of crime for profit and ways of tackling it*. Oisterwijk, NL: Wolf Legal Publishers

Lega Nord (2018) Vaccini: Salvini, nessun obbligo per genitori che devono conoscere rischi e vantaggi. Available at: www.leganord.org/notizie/news-2018/16408-vaccini-salvini-nessun-obbligo-per-genitori-che-devono-conoscere-rischi-e-vantaggi

Lupia A (2013) Communicating science in politicized environments. *Proceedings of the National Academy of Sciences* 110(3):14048–1454

Ministero della Salute (2019) *I dati nazionali al 2017 sulle coperture vaccinali dell'età pediatrica e dell'adolescente*. Available at: www.salute.gov.it/portale/news/p3_2_1_1_1.jsp? lingua=italiano&menu=notizie&p=dalministero&id=3348

Mudde C (2004) The populist zeitgeist. *Government & Opposition* 39(3):541–563

Murthy D (2008) Digital ethnography: an examination of the use of new technologies for social research. *Sociology* 42(5):837–855

New York Times (2019) Trump tells Americans: 'go get your measles vaccination. Apr 26. Available at: www.nytimes.com/reuters/2019/04/26/us/26reuters-usa-measles-trump.html

Nicholson SP and Segura GM (2012) Who's the party of the people? Economic populism and the US public's beliefs about political parties. *Political Behavior* 34(2):369–389

Nisbet MC and Huge M (2006) Attention cycles and frames in the plant biotechnology debate: managing power and participation through the press/policy connection. *Harvard International Journal of Press* 8(2):36–70

Osservatorio Scienza Tecnologia e Società (2017) Italiani e vaccini: i nuovi dati dell'Osservatorio. Available at: www.observa.it/italiani-e-vaccini-i-nuovi-dati-dellosservatorio/

Paun C (2017) *Trump offers vindication to vaccine skeptic doctor*. Available at: www.politico.eu/article/disgraced-doctor-who-questioned-vaccine-safetylooks-to-trump-with-hope/

Pink S, Horst H, Postill J, Hjorth L, Lewis T and Tacchi J (2016) *Digital ethnography: principles and practice*. London: Sage

Roberts M (2016) *The long depression*. Chicago: Haymarket

Roux C and Verzichelli L (2010) Still a pro-European but not a fully Europeanised elite? *South European Society and Politics* 15(1):11–33

Rovira Kaltwasser C (2015) Explaining the emergence of populism in Europe and the Americas. In De la Torre C (ed.) *The promise and perils of populism*. Lexington, KY: University Press of Kentucky

Serricchio F (2012) Italian citizens and Europe: explaining the growth of Euroscepticism. *Bulletin of Italian Politics* 4(1):115–134

Taber CS and Lodge M (2006) Motivated skepticism in the evaluation of political beliefs. *American Journal of Political Science* 50(3):755–789

Trump D (2018) *Lesley Stahl interviews Donald Trump on 60 minutes*. Oct 14. Available at: https://factba.se/transcript/donald-trump-interview-60-minutes-october-14-2018

US Preventive Services Task Force (USPSTF) (2009) Screening for breast cancer: US preventive services task force recommendation statement. *Annals of Internal Medicine* 151(10):716–726

Wakefield AJ, Murch SH, Anthony A, Linnell J, Casson DM, Malik M, Dhillon AP, Thomson MA, Harvey P, Valentine A, Davies SE and Walker-Smith JE (1998) Ileal-lymphoid-nodular hyperplasia, non-specific colitis, and pervasive developmental disorder in children. *Lancet* 351:637–641

WHO (2017) WHO-UNICEF coverage estimates. Available at: http://apps.who.int/immunization_monitoring/globalsummary/timeseries/tscove ragemcv1.html

WHO (2018) 10 Facts on immunization. Available at: www.who.int/features/factfiles/immunization/en

7 Quantum physics and the modern trends in pseudoscience

Enrico Gazzola

Introduction

In pseudoscientific arguments, quantum physics (hereafter QP) is often mentioned as a way to provide foundations to unrelated or absurd claims related to new-age spiritual doctrines, dubious medical practices, or different kinds of commercial products. Various beliefs or superstitions are claimed to be consequences of QP, for example the ideas that the human mind controls and creates the material world, that people can be telepathically connected, that our bodies or souls are made of energy, that diseases are a consequence of some energetic field imbalance, or that remote healing is possible (Redwood 1995; Landau 2011; Walia 2014; Lubbock 2017; Montana 2017; Jurgan 2018). The subtle use of fake scientific foundations is an established strategy used by 'quacks' to promote their ideas and try to convince their customers, and sometimes even medical professionals, of their validity. By exhibiting a collection of logical fallacies, their approach usually includes anecdotal reports, (often famous) testimonials, conspiracy accusations against the scientific mainstream, and appeals to 'nature' and ancient wisdom, but also references to cutting-edge science (Novella 2014).

Quacks seem to despise science, but they also want to mimic and resemble it in order to seize its prestige and reliability in the eyes of the customer, despite actually lacking any scientific methodology and therefore resulting in a parody (Beyerstein 1995). If the aim is to fool the customer, invoking advanced and not widely understood scientific concepts may be a winning strategy. Indeed, QP is such a complex and deeply unfamiliar subject that—when embedded in an argument—the average customer, although sceptical, would have a hard time dismissing it; in addition, QP is well known for actually being weird and predicting incredible phenomena. Consider, for instance, the existence of private associations (which present themselves as 'academies' or 'universities') promoting the inclusion of quantum quackeries in alternative medicine practices.[1] These 'academies' take the appearance of educational institutions, offering questionable certifications and degrees, while presenting pseudoscientific practices of the like of 'quantum medicine', 'quantum healing', or 'quantum homeopathy' as if they were legitimate medical practices. Of course, these associations are not recognised as universities and their courses and degrees are not accredited by the proper national education authorities. However, they are recognised by some national and international organisations of alternative and naturopathic medicine.[2]

Actual QP, however, is not a magical justification for unscientific claims. On the contrary, most statements flaunted in 'alternative' currents are in clear conflict with well-established physical laws. For these reasons, this chapter is devoted to identifying, understanding, and dismissing quantum quackery by briefly clarifying what QP actually is and what it is not and some typical related scams. Some fundamental concepts will be introduced together with their most relevant and widespread misconceptions. We will review common tactics of pseudoscience based on abuse of scientific terminology, and examine how certain 'alternative' medical practices are built on nonsensical statements and technobabble. We will also encounter some cases in which unfounded claims are based on controversial or dismissed physical models. These cases are complex, as the quackery is based on a sophisticated formal background, which can be effectively dismissed only by those with disciplinary expertise.

Quantum physics and its misconceptions

QP has been a major scientific, cultural, and technological revolution and is today one of the central theories of modern physics. At the beginning of the 20th century, the experimental capability to investigate the microscopic structure of matter produced a set of results that required a radical paradigm change to be explained (Jammer 1966; Omnès 1999). QP was therefore developed, starting as a collection of ad hoc models and then evolving into a full formal theory of the microscopic world (where by 'theory' we mean a mathematical model which provides some knowledge about the world, allowing to explain and predict phenomena). Specifically, QP is the theory which investigates the structure and behaviour of matter and light at a microscopic level. In other words, it describes the dynamics of molecules, atoms, and subatomic particles, and also of the light at the scale at which individual indivisible 'packets' of light (photons) are identified. QP is also needed to understand phenomena involving slightly bigger systems, if those are kept at a temperature close to absolute zero—these are known as 'ultracold' systems (Bloch et al. 2012; Madison et al. 2015). QP is nowadays a well-established theory, rooted in experiment. It provides technological applications, including laser, microelectronics (which make our computers and smartphones work), photovoltaic panels, and all the nuclear physics-based technologies (with medical imaging like NMR and PET among them) (Matson 2010; Orzel 2015). An emerging new generation of quantum technologies is attracting great interest and big investments in the information and communication technologies and metrology fields (Dowling and Milburn 2003; Allen 2016).

QP is a fascinating yet counterintuitive and profoundly complicated topic: it is at odds with the teachings of previous physical theories (now called 'classical physics') and contradicts any 'common sense'. While generations of physicists studied and grasped its principles and applications, its spreading in popular culture is affected by remarkable misunderstandings and confusion, both accidental and fraudulent (Gardner and Wheeler 1979; Gell-Mann 1995; Stenger 1997; Boyle 2010). Consequently, many tend to associate 'quantum physics' with quite anything that comes to their minds, mixing badly understood concepts from physics with their personal beliefs.

This situation has historical precedents. For instance, there was an age when magnetism (i.e., a class of physical phenomena mediated by magnetic field) was still a quite mysterious thing and as such subject to misunderstanding and quackeries. In the 18th century, for instance, the German doctor Franz Mesmer introduced the hypothesis of 'animal magnetism'. For 'animal magnetism', Dr Mesmer intended a universal natural force in the form of an invisible fluid flowing in living beings and capable of physical effects, including healing illness (Darnton 1968). Mesmer's claims were the object of a formal investigation held by a Royal Commission appointed in Paris in 1784 and run by prominent scientists such as Benjamin Franklin and Antoine Lavoisier. During this investigation, blind trials (which are now a common methodology in clinical research) were used as a way to assess suspicious practices for the first time (Kaptchuk 1998). Some of the ideas derived by the animal magnetism hypothesis may sound hilarious today—for instance, a French occultist in the 19th century proposed an instant communication machine based on 'telepathic' snails (Rosen 2016). We can state today that magnetism would not produce this type of phenomena, because it rigorously obeys a certain—and very different—set of physical laws. This is still true also for QP. While magnetism-based pseudoscientific ideas are no longer in fashion nowadays, quantum-based ones are thriving and increasingly producing unexpected nonsense and 'disciplines' as diverse as 'quantum agriculture' (*NewScientist* 2013; Wright et al. 2017), 'quantum nutrition' (Schwarcz 2017), and even 'quantum beauty/cosmetology' (ElCoin 2018). To physicists, those 'disciplines' sound as hilarious as Mesmer's ideas. Through logical fallacies and lexical ambiguities, physics jargon is distorted to evoke implausible scientific arguments and support wrong claims, often related to health. This strategy has been exploited both by traditional forms of alternative treatments such as homeopathy or reiki (Gunter 2015; Walia 2016), and by new ones such as quantum medicine, energetic medicine, quantum healing, and theta healing (Landau 2011; *AsayaMind* 2016; Jurgan 2018).

The observer

One of the most misunderstood concepts is the role of so-called observer. In QP, the observation, or measurement, is an action aimed at determining the value of a property of a particle, like its position, velocity, polarisation, or else. According to QP, this property may not have a defined value before the measurement; furthermore, the outcome of a measurement is completely random among the set of possible outcomes. A widespread misunderstanding is that the 'observer' should be a conscious human being—a controversial idea initially proposed by some of the scientists who founded QP itself such as Heisenberg,

Schrödinger, and for some time Bohr, while many others such as Einstein, Planck, and De Broglie opposed it (Marin 2009; Zyga 2009). The idea of the human observer was ultimately dismissed as untenable. Therefore, we can now state that the observer is not a conscious human being, but rather any apparatus which can provide a univocal reading of the value of that property (Zeilinger 1999; Myrvold 2016). Nonetheless, the 'conscious observer' idea survived, being promoted and popularised by a group of young unemployed physicists devoted to a hippie lifestyle, who called themselves Fundamental Fysiks Group (Kaiser 2011; Schweber 2011). One of them, Fritjof Capra, became a notable reference for new-agers: he wrote the bestselling book *The Tao of Physics* (Capra 1975), providing debatable and often misleading parallels between QP and eastern mysticism (Scerri 1989; Lederman and Teresi 1993). Interestingly, while Fritjof Capra himself clarified that his comparison should not be taken literally, other popular new-age authors refer to him when arguing that modern physics is rediscovering ancient wisdom and that there are connections between QP and exotic philosophies (Malkowski 2008; Stenger 2014).

While the discussion about what precisely is an observer in QP is pretty much a philosophical issue, there is a further important fact to understand, whose negation is a clear step towards pseudoscience: the observer does not decide the result, it only forces the system to provide a result, namely to set the measured quantity on one precise value among the possible ones. The selection of the final value is an intrinsically random process; this is a peculiar fundamental property of QP. Denial of this fact is quite popular among new-age currents, because it provides the basis for a belief called 'the law of attraction'. According to the law of attraction, one can 'attract' his/her desires and have them fulfilled just by will. In her book *The Secret* (arguably the most widespread and popular book on the topic), Rhonda Byrne states that the universe is shaped by our thought and ascribes this claim to QP (Byrne 2006). To be clear, the so-called law of attraction is in no way a law of QP or physics in general, and the misuse Byrne (among others) makes of scientific concepts has been widely criticised (Shermer 2007; Radford 2009; Matson 2010; Randall 2011). The law of attraction is in fact physically untenable on many levels, as it requires a series of deceptive assumptions to be justified: (1) that the observation in QP needs to be the action of a human being; (2) that the observer can pilot the result of the measurement (thus having his/her desires fulfilled); and (3) that in this way the observer can magically pilot his/her own whole future. Of course, if someone is led to believe such a thing, he or she will also believe that such power could be used for healing purposes. It is easy to access anecdotal reports or instructions containing extraordinary claims about the power of the law of attraction to heal diseases, including very serious or incurable ones (Zink 2015; *TheWisdomPost* 2018). It is also interesting to note that according to the law of attraction we are also responsible for anything bad that happens to us, including accidents, diseases, and even death, because we attract them with our thoughts. By responsabilising (and putting the blame on) individuals for what happens to them, the law of attraction can always avoid admitting its failure, and therefore can shield any attempt to be methodically tested. In other words, since the law is perfect, the victim is to be blamed if it fails (Farber 2016).

QP is today commonly—yet inappropriately—invoked in support to this system of beliefs, which has to be considered a deceptive commercial strategy, lacking any scientific foundation.

Entanglement

Another major misconception is related to 'entanglement', which is arguably the most peculiar and mind-blowing phenomenon arising in QP. Entanglement is a very unusual kind of correlation between the values of some quantities (which may be, as before, position, velocity, polarisation, or others). Before presenting this phenomenon, we shall give a basic understanding of what a correlation is, by considering a pair of gloves. Let us imagine that Enrico takes a pair of gloves, puts the two gloves in two boxes, and sends one box to Anita and one box to Anna. When Anita opens her box and finds, for example, the right glove, she will instantly know that the other box, wherever it is, contains the left glove, because they came from a pair. It is clear that Anita gains this knowledge without any communication with Anna, and that in no way could she send a message to Anna through the gloves. From this example, we can make two statements. First, there is a correlation between the handedness of the gloves; therefore, it is sufficient to open one box to know the content of both boxes (in one there will be the left glove, and in the other the right glove). Second, the matching of gloves with boxes is determined from the beginning, at the moment when Enrico puts them into the boxes. It may appear pointless to separate these two statements, but when it comes to entanglement their separation becomes relevant, as only one of the two holds true. As firstly demonstrated in a milestone paper by Einstein, Podolsky, and Rosen (Einstein et al. 1935) and successively proved in countless experiments (Zeilinger 1999), QP offers the possibility to prepare particles in a particular kind of correlated state, quite like the two gloves in the example above, yet with a crucial difference. Without entering too much into details, we may say that if our gloves were quantum particles and their handedness a quantum property, our second statement (i.e., that the handedness of each was already fixed from the beginning) may not hold true. While our first statement still holds (there is a correlation, meaning that it is sufficient to determine the handedness of a quantum glove to fix also the handedness of the other), we are forced to accept that which glove was in which box will only be determined when one of the boxes is opened. Whatever the distance between the two correlated quantum gloves, the measure of the handedness of one also determines the handedness of the other. It is still a form of correlation, but of a kind that only holds at the scale where quantum rules hold—this is what is called quantum entanglement.

Not surprisingly, this concept suffers widespread misunderstandings. It is also very much used by 'quacks' to support fantastic claims—like the existence of entanglement between brains or people allowing such things as telepathic connections and healing at a distance to happen (Milgrom 2007, 2008; Tressoldi et al. 2010; Erickson 2011; Rabyor 2014; Jurgan 2018). An extreme case is that of the QuantumMAN website ('closed for improvements' for some time now). The website advertised 'the first downloadable medicine', selling alleged medical treatments (ranging from quantum massage to the malaria vaccine) in the form of files to be downloaded to a pc or mobile phone from where they would *quantistically* act on the patient's body through entanglement and teleportation (Gorski 2012a, b; Carroll and Renish 2013). The idea of a relation between entanglement, telepathy, and teleportation is common only in a certain faction of paranormal investigators: the ones who do not actually know QP (those with background knowledge in physics are aware that entanglement in this context can be considered only as a metaphor, see Bem 2011). The main misunderstanding here has to do with wrongly associating entanglement with some kind of instantaneous communication between the two entangled particles. This would be like saying that Anita could send Anna a message by modifying the handedness of her quantum glove, resulting in a correspondent instantaneous modification of the other. This is completely wrong because Anita cannot decide the handedness of her glove: according to QP, she can only fix it by a measurement, whose result will be absolutely random between the two possible results (Bruss et al. 2000). This action will correspondingly fix also the handedness of Anna's glove, but this does not mean that the glove will switch from a determined handedness to another; rather, it will pass from an undetermined handedness to a determined one. Anna cannot, by any means, detect any difference produced by Anita's action, because she cannot monitor the glove handedness: she can only measure it at a certain moment in time.

In order to dismiss most pseudoscientific claims about entanglement, we should remember that entanglement is neither an instantaneous, slow, nor fast form of communication. In fact, it is not a communication at all. Also, it is not an unbreakable bond; on the contrary, it is a very ephemeral condition, that is terminated by the measurement (after the handedness of the two quantum gloves is determined, they are not in entanglement anymore and subsequent actions on one glove will have no effect on the other) or broken by random interactions with the environment. Finally, entanglement is a condition which can be achieved only in the quantum realm (i.e., microscopic or ultracold systems) and maintained for short times by accurate experimental set-ups.

Lexical ambiguities

It is a common feature of pseudoscientific arguments to use obscure and impressive statements which may seem profound but are actually meaningless. These kinds of statements have been labelled by some authors 'pseudo-profound bullshit' (Pennycook et al. 2015, 2016), with a definition which distinguishes them by mere nonsense: while nonsense may be a collection of words just picked up randomly and lacking both illusory and actual meaning, 'pseudo-profound arguments' are presented with a syntactic structure that suggests that the sentence is intended to communicate something (possibly deep in meaning) despite being constructed in a way that is intentionally ambiguous and fundamentally vacuous. QP unfortunately offers easy ground to this strategy. A typical trick used by 'quacks' is to exploit the mismatch between the specific technical meaning of some terms in physics and the different or ambiguous meaning they assume in common language. For example, some common expressions, such as 'feeling/sending good vibration' or have 'positive energies', have a metaphoric meaning that is completely unrelated to the scientific terms 'vibration' (mechanical non-propagating oscillations), 'frequency' (the number of oscillations per second of a periodic phenomenon), or 'energy' (an abstract quantity associated to physical systems). In particular, a cartoonish interpretation of the concept of energy is widely diffused, with energy being imagined as a kind of cosmic entity with effects on health or destiny (Landau 2011; Walia 2014; Lubbock 2017; Montana 2017; Jurgan 2018). A relevant example is a (fake) quote attributed to Albert Einstein: 'Everything is energy and that's all there is to it. Match the frequency of the reality you want and you cannot help but get that reality. It can be no other way. This is not philosophy. This is physics'. These absurd statements could hardly have been made by Einstein. According to the website QuoteInvestigator, the quote probably comes from a spiritual 'guru', a promoter of healing meditation (O'Toole 2012). In addition, the already mentioned law of attraction often 'plays' with the definition of scientific concepts by claiming that energy vibrates at certain frequencies, and that people (being also made of energy) are also vibrating at their own frequencies, which resonate with the frequency of the universe (Byrne 2006). Of course, none of this has any sense in QP or in physics in general.

The idea that our bodies 'are made of energy', which was born as a popular misunderstanding of Einstein's mass-energy equivalence (Fernflores 2012), has quickly led to the idea that diseases are the result of some kind of imbalance in an alleged energetic field of the body, and that the cure should therefore be not chemical but 'energetic'. These ideas are at the basis of pseudoscientific practices such as energetic healing, quantum healing, and theta healing. In addition, also more established practices based on the idea that the body contains some non-physical 'energetic system' (like chakra healing, pranotherapy, and reiki) may be prone to this type of linguistic misconception.

A well-known master of quantum woo is the former physician Deepak Chopra, one of the most famous holistic healing advocates worldwide (Pennycook 2015). He coined the practice of 'quantum healing' by postulating a connection between QP and a deep level of consciousness, which he calls the 'quantum mechanical body' (Chopra 1989). In his practice, this level of consciousness is reached by individuals through meditation and visualisation, which allegedly result in the production by the body of an extraordinary healing capability, with the potential to defeat deadly diseases like cancer, or even aging itself (Horgan 2016) Among Chopra's claims falsely related to QP is that our bodies are fields of information and energy and that quantum healing would act through a 'shift in the fields of energy information' (Redwood

1995). Concepts such as 'field of information' or 'field of energy' make no sense in physics (where a 'field' is an extended entity identified by a value in each point of space, and 'energy' and 'information' are quantities carried by physical systems). Once again, scientific terms are used to blur the boundaries between the physical and the mystical worlds.

Quantum woo in practice

Homeopathy and the water memory

In the previous sections, we have seen that new (and most absurd) alternative practices emerge from a confusion on the fundamental principles of QP. However, alternative medical practices with a longstanding tradition also take advantage of this new quantum-related pseudoscientific trend. Homeopathy is among the most-known and -used alternative medical practices in the world, and it is based on remedies obtained by extreme dilution of active principles in solutions (Vickers and Zollman 1999). Since the discovery of chemistry, we know that homeopathic preparations are so diluted that almost no trace of the active principle is found in there anymore, thus precluding any chemical effect; also, worldwide clinical trials and meta-analyses have shown that homeopathic remedies have only placebo effects (Shang et al. 2005; Mashta 2009; Ernst 2010; Mathie et al. 2017). In the attempt to find a theoretical foundation to validate their approach, some homeopaths have started to involve QP-related 'explanations' (Schulte and Endler 2015; Almirantis and Tsitinidis 2018), for instance by claiming that through QP it would be possible to overcome the chemical impossibilities of homeopathy. Arguably the most famous of these attempts is related to the alleged 'water memory', a phenomenon reported by Benveniste in a controversial paper on *Nature* in 1988, according to which highly diluted human antibodies preserved their biological action (Davenas et al. 1988). The results were soon dismissed by attempts of replication (Maddox et al. 1988). Benveniste, however, never gave up the ideas presented in that paper. These ideas found further support by a new line of highly controversial research supported by Luc Montagnier, former Nobel Prize winner for the discovery of HIV. Unfortunately, Montagnier became also notorious for having embraced various unscientific positions, including claims about DNA 'teleportation' (Lowe 2011; Gorski 2011, 2012a, b). In a series of experiments published in 2009 in a new journal, *Interdisciplinary Sciences: Computational Life Sciences* (of which Montagnier was chair of the editorial board), Montagnier and colleagues reported low frequency electromagnetic signals emission from DNA sequences in high aqueous dilution, and associated them to the formation of water nanostructures (Montagnier et al. 2009a, b). Allegedly, the nanostructures recreated by the electromagnetic signals in a different recipient containing only pure water would be 'recognised' by DNA replication enzymes. Hence, DNA sequences could be recreated by their imprint on water (Montagnier et al. 2011, 2015). Montagnier's results, however, were largely ignored by the scientific community (Coghlan 2011; *NewScientist* 2011; Ball 2013) because of the raw methods used, the unreasonable claims done in relation to the results, and the bad presentation of the results themselves. Nonetheless, these results, including the water memory, are still largely cited by homeopathy's advocates, as they seem to support the idea that something may still happen at high dilution (Enserink 2010; Grimes 2012). Moreover, the fact that Montagnier is a former Nobel Prize winner is often mentioned to imply the credibility of his idea towards non-experts.

QP came into play when Montagnier's claims met the ideas carried forward by a group of Italian physicists, most notably Giuliano Preparata and Emilio del Giudice. After a high-profile career in particle physics, Preparata, together with his disciple Del Giudice, developed a model predicting large-scale quantum phenomena in matter (Biazzo and Garra 2010; Liberti 2010). According to this model, relatively big regions (called 'coherence domains') where quantum rules hold can be found in some materials, in particular in water (Preparata 1995). Successive research never found evidence of these coherence domains, and Preparata's model fell into the circle of failed theoretical attempts. Unfortunately, Preparata never accepted to dismiss his model and, in the absence of legitimate experimental results to support it, he turned to controversial ones such as cold fusion (which postulates that nuclear fusion could occur in materials at room temperature) and the above-mentioned memory of water (Preparata et al. 1989; Del Giudice and Preparata 1998). Although Preparata's model has substantially been forgotten by the scientific community, it still survives in dubious and pseudoscientific research streams. For instance, Preparata's model is invoked in support of the idea that the electromagnetic field regulates and coordinates human cells at a long range (a hypothesis suggesting the possibility to heal diseases by regulating the field through a machine, a plate, able to 'inform' water (Sermoneta 2016)). Interestingly, the concept of the 'informed water' is out of the boundaries of Preparata's model, that is here merely exploited to build a technobabble to justify the sale of the machine. The name and questionable ideas of former high-profile scientists is exploited to make a commercial operation more insidious and more difficult to recognise as a pseudoscientific practice by inexperienced customers.

The Nelson case

Confiding in alternative medical practices while refusing conventional treatments often has a tragic impact on the health and wellbeing of individuals, even leading to their premature death (Han et al. 2011; Joseph et al. 2012; Saquib et al. 2012; Johnson et al. 2018). Despite the significant harm that we can expect from many quantum-related quackeries, juridical cases specifically focused on them can hardly be found, and therefore the dark number of victims remains high. This is probably because quantum woo, as we presented it above, generally does not stand on its own in the field of alternative medical practices; quantum woo can be better interpreted as an umbrella approach, exploited by many pseudoscientific streams to cover their unscientific thinking with a cape of complicated and apparently scientific concepts, in order to make it more difficult to unravel, recognise, and oppose their fabrications.

One the boldest healthcare frauds based on a quantum-based medical scam is the *Quantum Biofeedback* case, orchestrated by William Nelson.[3] Back in 2007, a *Seattle Times* investigation reported a worldwide network of manufacturers, sellers, and practitioners of non-scientific medical devices and practices (Willmsen and Berens 2007). According to the inquiry, for decades Nelson sold in the United States a machine called EPFX, claiming it was capable of diagnosing any disease (including AIDS and cancer) and of removing it with an electromagnetic 'zap'. Mr Nelson registered his company with the Food and Drug Administration as a producer of biofeedback machines (i.e., stress-relieving devices). In 1996, after being charged of felony fraud, he fled the country but never stopped running his business from his new headquarters in Budapest. Quite the opposite, he commercialised an 'improved' version of the machine called Quantum Xrroid Interface System, using a greater level of quantum woo in its marketing (Barrett 2009). The *Seattle Times* estimated that more than 10,000 devices were sold in the United States alone (including in a hospital) because of the belief that these machines could substitute legit medical treatments (a belief partially supported by the fact that Nelson's company was registered with the FDA, which was not aware of the diffusion and actual use of the above-mentioned machines).

Concluding remarks

There is agreement in the scientific community that medical treatments do not need a complete explanation of their working mechanisms as long as they can be proved effective with clinical evidence. Scientific research is by definition open-minded. But being open to what is new does not mean that we should uncritically accept health practices that base their marketing on pseudoscientific arguments, especially if those arguments are used to prevent scientific verification of the clinical effects of such health practices. Unfortunately, the highly complex and deeply counterintuitive nature of QP provides fertile ground for false experts and fraudsters, with quantum-inspired woo fitting their strategy of stealing and distorting concepts from science in order to produce fake scientific foundations to absurd claims. QP does not support claims concerning mystical energies, healing frequencies, energetic patterns in the body, creating thoughts, universal consciousness, or the existence of the soul. While QP has indeed a role in imaging technologies with medical applications (like NMR), no healing practice can be expected to be directly related to it.

Notes

1 Consider, for instance, www.qfa-aaqm.org/ and quantumuniversity.com/.
2 As reported, for instance, in quantumuniversity.com/how-it-works/#accreditation.
3 US District Court, District of Columbia (Washington, DC) No.1:96-cr-00209–1.

References

Allen M (2016) Physicists release 'quantum manifesto' for Europe. *Physics World* 29(4):10

Almirantis Y and Tsitinidis K (2018) Ultra-high dilutions and homeopathy: can they be explained without non-local theory? *Homeopathy* 107(3):189–195

AsayaMind (2016) Energy healing – Using applied quantum physics to transform any area of your life. *Asayamind*. Mar 6. Available at: https://asayamind.com/energy-healing-using-applied-quantum-physics-to-transform-any-area-of-your-life/

Ball P (2013) DNA waves don't wash. *Chemistry World*. Jul 10. Available at: www.chemistry-world.com/opinion/dna-waves-dont-wash/6373.article

Barrett S (2009) Some notes on the Quantum Xrroid (QXCI) and William C. Nelson. *Quack Watch* [online]. Jul 12. Available at: www.quackwatch.org/01QuackeryRelatedTopics/Tests/xrroid.html

Bem DJ (2011) Feeling the future: experimental evidence for anomalous retroactive influences on cognition and affect. *Journal of Personality and Social Psychology* 100(3):407–425

Beyerstein BL (1995) Distinguishing science from pseudoscience. Victoria, BC: The Centre for Curriculum and Professional Development

Biazzo I and Garra R (2010) Dai quark ai cristalli: quarant'anni di storia della fisica attraverso gli occhi di Giuliano Preparata. *Accastampato* 3(7)

Bloch I, Dalibard J and Nascimbène S (2012) Quantum simulations with ultracold quantum gases. *Nature Physics* 8(4):267–276

Boyle A (2010) How to spot quantum quackery. *NCB News*. Sep 20. Available at: www.nbcnews.com/science/how-spot-quantum-quackery-6C10403763

Bruss D, D'Ariano GM, Macchiavello C and Sacchi MF (2000) Approximate quantum cloning and the impossibility of superluminal information transfer. *Physical Review A* 62:062302

Byrne R (2006) *The Secret*. New York: Atria

Capra F (1975) *The tao of physics*. Boulder, CO: Shambhala

Carroll B and Renish J (2013) QuantumMan's downloadable medicine & extraterrestrial technology. *The Skeptic's Dictionary Newsletter* 12(2)

Chopra D (1989) *Quantum healing: exploring the frontiers of mind/body medicine*. New York: Bantam

Coghlan A (2011) Scorn over claim of teleported DNA. *NewScientist*. Jan 12. Available at: www.newscientist.com/article/mg20927952-900-scorn-over-claim-of-teleported-dna

Darnton R (1968) *Mesmerism and the end of the enlightenment*. Cambridge, MA: Harvard University Press

Davenas E, Beauvais F, Amara J, Oberbaum M, Robinzon B, Miadonnai A, Tedeschi A, Pomeranz B, Fortner P, Belon P, Sainte-Laudy J, Poitevin B and Benveniste J (1988) Human basophil degranulation triggered by very dilute antiserum against IgE. *Nature* 333(6176):816–818

Del Giudice E and Preparata G (1998) Coherent electrodynamics in water. In Sculte J and Endler C (eds.) *Fundamental research in ultrahigh dilution and homeopathy*. Dordrecht, The Netherlands: Kluwer

Dowling JP and Milburn GJ (2003) Quantum technology: the second quantum revolution. *Philosophical Transactions of the Royal Society of London A* 361:1655–1674

Einstein A, Podolsky B and Rosen N (1935) Can quantum-mechanical description of physical reality be considered complete? *Physical Review* 47:777–780

ElCoin (2018) Quantum cosmetology device is ready. *Medium*. Apr 17. Available at: https://medium.com/@ELCoin/quantum-cosmetology-device-is-ready-9374e771dfaa

Enserink M (2010) French Nobelist escapes 'intellectual terror' to pursue radical ideas in China. *Science* 330(6012):1732

Erickson DL (2011) Intuition, telepathy, and interspecies communication. *NeuroQuantology* 9(1):145–152

Ernst E (2010) Homeopathy: what does the 'best' evidence tell us? *The Medical Journal of Australia* 192(8):458–460

Farber N (2016) The truth about the law of attraction. *Psychology Today*. Sept 18. Available at: www.psychologytoday.com/us/blog/the-blame-game/201609/the-truth-about-the-law-attraction

Fernflores F (2012) The equivalence of mass and energy. *The Stanford Encyclopedia of Philosophy* (Spring 2012 Edition). Available at: plato.stanford.edu/entries/equivME/

Gardner M and Wheeler JA (1979) Quantum theory and quack theory. *The New York Review of Books*. May 17, 40–41. Available at: www.nybooks.com/articles/1979/05/17/quantum-theory-and-quack-theory/

Gell-Mann M (1995) *The Quark and the Jaguar: adventures in the simple and the complex*. New York: Freeman

Gorski D (2011) The Nobel disease meets DNA teleportation and homeopathy. *Respectful Insolence*. Jan 14. Available at: https://scienceblogs.com/insolence/2011/01/14/the-nobel-disease-meets-dna-teleportatio

Gorski D (2012a) Closing out 2012 with a bit of fun: do you want some quantum with that pseudoscience? *Science-based Medicine*. Dec 31. Available at: https://sciencebasedmedicine.org/do-you-want-some-quantum-with-that-pseudoscience/

Gorski D (2012b) Luc Montagnier and the Nobel Disease. *Science-based Medicine*. Jun 4. Available at: https://sciencebasedmedicine.org/luc-montagnier-and-the-nobel-disease/

Grimes DR (2012) Proposed mechanisms for homeopathy are physically impossible. *Focus on Alternative and Complementary Therapies* 17(3):149–155

Gunter J (2015) Can quantum mechanics explain homeopathy? *Dr Jen Gunter*. Jul 9. Available at: https://drjengunter.wordpress.com/2015/07/09/can-quantum-mechanics-explain-homeopathy/

Han E, Johnson N, DelaMelena T, Glissmeyer M and Steinbock K (2011) Alternative therapy used as primary treatment for breast cancer negatively impacts outcomes. *Annals of Surgical Oncology* 18(4):912–916

Horgan J (2016) My doubts about Deepak Chopra and the monetization of meditation. *Scientific American*. Sept 19. Available at: https://blogs.scientificamerican.com/cross-check/my-doubts-about-deepak-chopra-and-the-monetization-of-meditation/

Jammer M (1966) *The conceptual development of quantum mechanics*. New York: McGraw-Hill

Johnson SB, Park HS, Gross CP and Yu JB (2018) Use of alternative medicine for cancer and its impact on survival. *Journal of the National Cancer Institute* 110(1):121–124

Joseph K, Vrouwe S, Kamruzzaman A, Balbaid A, Fenton D, Berendt R, Yu E and Tai P (2012) Outcome analysis of breast cancer patients who declined evidence-based treatment. *World Journal of Surgical Oncology* 10(118)

Jurgan J (2018) Why distant healing works and is more powerful than you think. *Blossom of the soul*. May 24. Available at: www.blossomofthesoul.org/2018/05/24/why-distant-healing-works-and-is-more-powerful-than-you-think/

Kaiser D (2011) *How the hippies saved physics*. New York: W.W. Norton & Co

Kaptchuk TJ (1998) Intentional ignorance: a history of bind assessment and placebo controls in medicine. *Bulletin of the History of Medicine* 72(3):389–433

Landau MD (2011) Energy healed me – over the phone! A scientist explains how. *Huffington Post*. Oct. 19. Available at: www.huffpost.com/entry/healing-over-the-phone_b_1011510

Lederman L and Teresi D (1993) *The God particle: if the Universe is the answer, what is the question?* New York: Delta

Liberti P (2010) Giuliano Preparata, le molte vite di un uomo singolare. *Query*. Dec 10. Available at: www.queryonline.it/2010/12/10/giuliano-preparata-le-molte-vite-di-un-uomo-singolare/

Lowe D (2011) Has Luc Montagnier lost it? *In the Pipeline*. Jan 10. Available at: https://blogs.sciencemag.org/pipeline/archives/2011/01/10/has_luc_montagnier_lost_it

Lubbock P (2017) The science of energy medicine: how to work with subtle energy for better health. *Conscious Lifestyle Magazine*. Available at: www.consciouslifestylemag.com/energy-medicine-guide/

Maddox J, Randi J and Stewart WW (1988) 'High-dilution' experiments a delusion. *Nature* 334:287–291

Madison KW, Bongs K, Wang YQ, Rey AM and Zhai H (eds.) (2015) *Annual review of cold atoms and molecules*, vol. 3. Singapore: World Scientific

Malkowski EF (2008) Quantum philosophy and the ancient mystery school, today's new science philosophy – old or new? *Graham Hancock*. Apr 17. Available at: https://grahamhancock.com/malkowskie1/

Marin JM (2009) 'Mysticism' in quantum mechanics: the forgotten controversy. *European Journal of Physics* 30:807–822

Mashta O (2009) WHO warns against using homoeopathy to treat serious diseases. *The British Medical Journal* 339:b3447

Mathie RT, Ramparsad N, Legg LA, Clausen J, Moss S, Davidson JRT, Messow CM and McConnachie A (2017) Randomised double-blind, placebo-controlled trials of non-individualised homeopathic treatment: systematic review and meta-analysis. *Systematic Reviews* 6(1):63

Matson J (2010) What is quantum mechanics good for? *Scientific American*. Nov 2. Available at: www.scientificamerican.com/article/everyday-quantum-physics/

Milgrom LR (2007) Journeys in the country of the blind: entanglement theory and the effects of blinding on trials of homeopathy and homeopathic provings. *Evidence-Based Complementary and Alternative Medicine* 4(1):7–16

Milgrom LR (2008) A new geometrical description of entanglement and the curative homeopathic process. *Journal of Alternative and Complementary Medicine* 14(3):329–339

Montagnier L, Aïssa J, Del Giudice E, Lavallée C, Tedeschi A and Vitiello G (2011) DNA waves and water. *Journal of Physics: Conference Series* 306:012007

Montagnier L, Aïssa J, Ferris S, Montagnier JL and Lavallée C (2009a) Electromagnetic signals are produced by aqueous nanostructures derived from bacterial DNA sequences. *Interdisciplinary Sciences, Computational Life Sciences* 1(2):81–90

Montagnier L, Aïssa J, Lavallée C, Mbamy M, Varon J and Chenal H (2009b) Electromagnetic detection of HIV DNA in the blood of AIDS patients treated by antiretroviral therapy. *Interdisciplinary Sciences: Computational Life Sciences* 1(4):245–253

Montagnier L, Del Giudice E, Aïssa J, Lavallée C, Motschwiller S, Capolupo A, Polcari A, Romano P, Tedeschi A and Vitiello G (2015) Transduction of DNA information through water and electromagnetic waves. *Electromagnetic Biology and Medicine* 34(2):106–112

Montana C (2017) The illusion of reality: the scientific proof that everything is energy and reality isn't real. *Conscious Lifestyle Magazine*. Available at: www.consciouslifestylemag.com/everything-is-energy-illusion-reality/

Myrvold W (2016) Philosophical issues in quantum theory. *Stanford Encyclopedia of Philosophy*. Jul 25. Available at: https://plato.stanford.edu/entries/qt-issues/

NewScientist (2011) Why we have to teleport disbelief. *NewScientist*. Jan 12. Available at: www.newscientist.com/article/mg20927951-900-why-we-have-to-teleport-disbelief/

NewScientist (2013) What would quantum agriculture be? *NewScientist.* 11 Dec. Available at: www.newscientist.com/article/mg22029471-300-feedback-what-would-quantum-agriculture-be/

Novella S (2014) Quantum snake oil – a primer. *Science-Based Medicine.* Jan 15. Available at: https://sciencebasedmedicine.org/quantum-snake-oil-a-primer/

Omnès R (1999) *Understanding quantum mechanics.* Princeton: Princeton University Press

Orzel C (2015) What has quantum mechanics ever done for us? *Forbes.* Aug 13. Available at: www.forbes.com/sites/chadorzel/2015/08/13/what-has-quantum-mechanics-ever-done-for-us/

O'Toole G (2012) Everything is energy and that's all there is to it. Match the frequency of the reality you want. *Quote Investigator.* May 16. Available at: https://quoteinvestigator.com/2012/05/16/everything-energy/

Pennycook G, Cheyne JA, Barr N, Koehler DJ and Fugelsang JA (2015) On the reception and detection of pseudo-profound bullshit. *Judgment and Decision Making* 10(6):549–563

Pennycook G, Cheyne JA, Barr N, Koehler DJ and Fugelsang JA (2016) It's still bullshit: reply to Dalton. *Judgment and Decision Making* 11:123–125

Preparata G (1995) *QED coherence in matter.* Singapore: World Scientific

Preparata G, Bressani T and Del Giudice E (1989) First steps towards an understanding of cold fusion. *Il Nuovo Cimento* 101(5):845–849

Rabyor B (2014) Distance healing is a form of quantum entanglement. *Phoenix Tools.* Apr 12. Available at: https://phoenixtools.org/distance-healing-form-quantum-entanglement/

Radford B (2009) The pseudoscience of 'the secret'. *Live Science.* Feb 3. Available at: www.livescience.com/5303-pseudoscience-secret.html

Randall L (2011) *Knocking on heaven's door: how physics and scientific thinking illuminate the universe and the modern world.* New York: Harper Collins

Redwood D (1995) Interviews with people who make a difference: quantum healing. *Healthy.net.* Available at: www.healthy.net/scr/interview.aspx?Id=167

Rosen R (2016) Psychic snail sex couldn't replace the telegraph, but one Frenchman sure tried. *Atlas Obscura.* May 12. Available at: www.atlasobscura.com/articles/psychic-snail-sex-couldnt-replace-the-telegraph-but-one-frenchman-sure-tried

Saquib J, Parker BA, Natarajan L, Madlensky L, Saquib N, Patterson RE, Newman VA and Pierce JP (2012) Prognosis following the use of complementary and alternative medicine in women diagnosed with breast cancer. *Complementary Therapies in Medicine* 20(5):283–290

Scerri ER (1989) Eastern mysticism and the alleged parallels with physics. *American Journal of Physics* 57:687–692

Schulte J and Endler PC (2015) Update on preliminary elements of a theory of ultra high dilutions. *Homeopathy* 104(4):337–342

Schwarcz J (2017) Nutrients with the right 'resonance frequency'. *McGill.* Mar 20. Available at: www.mcgill.ca/oss/article/health-supplements/nutrients-right-resonance-frequency

Schweber S (2011) Freewheeling fundamental physics. *Physics Today* 64(9):59–60

Sermoneta E (2016) Gocce sulla pelle. *Scienza e Conoscenza.* Jan 1. Available at: www.scienzaeconoscenza.it/blog/memoria_acqua/gocce-sulla-pelle

Shang A, Huwiler-Müntener K, Nartey L, Jüni P, Dörig S, Sterne JAC, Pewsner D and Egger M (2005) Are the clinical effects of homoeopathy placebo effects? Comparative study of placebo-controlled trials of homoeopathy and allopathy. *The Lancet* 366(9487):726–732

Shermer M (2007) The (other) secret. *Scientific American.* Jun 1. Available at: www.scientificamerican.com/article/the-other-secret

Stenger V (1997) Quantum quackery. *Skeptical Inquirer.* Jan 21. Available at: www.csicop.org/si/show/quantum_quackery

Stenger V (2014) The revolution that didn't happen. *Huffington Post*. Jul 18. Available at: www.huffingtonpost.com/victor-stenger/the-revolution-that-didnt_b_5600647.html

TheWisdomPost (2018) How to use law of attraction to cure serious diseases. *The Wisdom Post*. Available at: www.thewisdompost.com/law-of-attraction/how-to-use-law-of-attraction-to-cure-serious-diseases/1794

Tressoldi P, Storm L and Radin D (2010) Extrasensory perception and quantum models of cognition. *NeuroQuantology* 8(4):S81–S87

Vickers A and Zollman C (1999) ABC of complementary medicine: homoeopathy. *The British Medical Journal* 319:1115–1118

Walia A (2014) Nothing is solid and everything is energy – scientists explain the world of quantum physics. *Collective Evolution*. Sept 27. Available at: www.collective-evolution.com/2014/09/27/this-is-the-world-of-quantum-physics-nothing-is-solid-and-everything-is-energy/

Walia A (2016) How reiki actually works (the science part). *Collective Evolution*. Mar 11. Available at: www.collective-evolution.com/2016/03/11/how-reiki-actually-works-the-science-part/

Willmsen C and Berens MJ (2007) How one man's invention is part of a growing worldwide scam that snares the desperately ill. *The Seattle Times*. Nov 18. Available at: www.seattletimes.com/seattle-news/how-one-mans-invention-is-part-of-a-growing-worldwide-scam-that-snares-the-desperately-ill/

Wright J, Kieft H and von Diest S (2017) Quantum-based agriculture: the final frontier. Innovative research for organic 3.0. *Proceedings of the scientific track at the organic world congress 2017*, Nov 9–11 in Delhi, India

Zeilinger A (1999) Experiment and the foundations of quantum physics. *Reviews of Modern Physics* 71(2):S288–S297

Zink R (2015) Success & failures in healing cancer. *Law of Attraction Solutions*. Jan 4. Available at: https://lawofattractionsolutions.com/success-failures-healing-cancer/

Zyga L (2009) Quantum mysticism: gone but not forgotten. *Phys.org*. Jun 8. Available at: https://phys.org/news/2009-06-quantum-mysticism-forgotten.html

8 Who are the experts?

Examining the online promotion of misleading and harmful nutrition information

Heather Horsburgh and David Barron

Introduction

Navigating the nutrition information environment is not an easy task. When one searches for nutrition information online, they are confronted with conflicting and sometimes dangerous messages. Whilst current official dietary guidelines in the United Kingdom stipulate that most of our daily food intake should come from fruit, vegetables, and starchy carbohydrates, and we should be consuming only small amounts of fish and red and processed meats (Public Health England 2016), there are many other voices communicating information that contradicts these official guidelines. For example, according to one of the most popular diet and exercise programmes provided on fitness website Bodybuilding.com,[1] one should consume 1.28 grams of protein per pound of lean body weight, and this protein should come from meat, egg whites, fish, and protein powders (some vegetarian options are provided). Thus, a person weighing 180 lbs with 20% body fat would have to consume 184 g of protein from the above protein sources—the equivalent of about six chicken breasts. Another more extreme example comes from one diet that proposes we should 'Eat 30 bananas a day for 30 days', which was a suggested nutritional programme offered by *Freelee the banana girl*, who has a substantial social media following and has described herself as a 'health YouTuber'. Freelee, receiving much criticism for the highly restrictive and controversial nutrition advice she offers, now promotes a 'raw till 4' diet, which suggests eating only raw food until 4 pm (Winter 2014; Rudd and House 2018).

These examples highlight the contradictory information and advice that people can be exposed to online, with some being much more extreme and controversial than others. Some of the nutrition information that people are exposed to is far from healthy, can be dangerous, and, unfortunately, is not a rare occurrence in the world of online personalities offering health and fitness advice to large audiences. The level of harm associated with nutrition misinformation will depend on the extent of the misinformation and the degree to which the misinformation develops into behaviour. Unfortunately, there are examples where extreme beliefs and behaviours regarding nutrition have led to death. In one such example, Jessica Ainscough, a 30-year-old female who referred to herself as the 'Wellness Warrior' on social media, opted to treat her rare form of cancer with Gerson Therapy, which involves a very strict diet of 13 glasses of fruit and vegetable smoothies per day and multiple daily coffee enemas. Ainscough also promoted the diet as a way to treat cancer via her social media platforms (Davey 2015). As a result of opting for Gerson Therapy instead of following the advice of her doctor, Ainscough died in 2015. Despite the tragic circumstances around Ainscough's death, 'The Gerson Therapy: The Proven Nutritional Program for Cancer and Other Illnesses' (Gerson and Walker 2001) is still available on Amazon and, as of 3 April 2019, has 116 reviews and has been rated 4.6 out of 5 stars.

The American Dietetic Association (ADA; now called the Academy of Nutrition and Dietetics or AND) have defined nutrition misinformation (NM) as consisting of

> erroneous, incomplete, or misleading information without any scientific basis at all. It can be disseminated naively or with malicious or self-serving intent (including to sell products or to gain attention). Food and nutrition misinformation may be harmful to a consumer's health and general well-being and includes food faddism, health fraud, and misdirected claims.
>
> (in Ayoob et al. 2002:601)

This definition is useful in that it indicates that NM can be communicated naively by people who are interested in—and may or may not trust—the information and want to share it, but can also be communicated with self-serving and sometimes malicious intent. Indeed, there are documented examples of where individuals have communicated NM with the intention of deliberately (fraudulently) misleading consumers. Belle Gibson is one such documented example. Belle Gibson claimed to have cured her own terminal brain cancer through diet and lifestyle, without the help of western medicine. Gibson started a blog to document her journey, which then turned into a business (*The Whole Pantry*), a book deal, and a phone app. In 2015, Gibson revealed that she fabricated the whole story and never had terminal brain cancer (Phillip 2015; Lavorgna and Sugiura 2018). The deliberately misleading and fraudulent information communicated by Gibson is clearly irresponsible in that it has the potential to encourage others to try to treat cancer without science-based evidence.

NM is not a new concept or one that only affects the online environment. Indeed, the ADA has regularly published their stance on food and NM for over 20 years (Ashley and Jarvis 1995; Wansink 2006), while many academics have discussed longstanding issues relating to food marketing and regulation in the offline environment (Nestle 2013; Tempels et al. 2017; Leon and Ken 2019). Nevertheless, there are certain aspects of the online environment that warrant a focused discussion of NM. For example, information creation and exchange in the Web 2.0 environment are different from the traditional media. Specifically, in the online world, two-way communication is possible and potentially anyone with an internet connection and some very basic tech skills can create and share nutrition information with very large audiences who can interact with each other (Ventola 2014; Ma and Atkin 2017). As will be discussed in this chapter, online environments allow companies and individuals to capitalise on sharing erroneous or incomplete information to the public, in the hope of achieving financial, professional, or personal gain.

The aim of this chapter is not to make simplified judgements about what is correct and incorrect nutrition information in online settings—to do so would be to make overly simplistic conclusions of complex nutrition literature, which is something we are being critical of in this chapter and is discussed later. Rather, in delineating the issue of NM by drawing on relevant psychological, public health, and social and life science literature, this chapter highlights how there are too many unqualified voices online advocating many different nutrition protocols, many of which lack scientific evidence. Overall, the present chapter uses examples to show that the problem of NM is not necessarily the inaccuracy of the communicated information (though it can be inaccurate); rather, it has to do with how the information is communicated, who is communicating it, the reasons for communicating it, and the consequences of communicating it. This chapter also highlights the many harms associated with NM and discusses possible methods of tackling the issue.

Nutrition misinformation in the online environment

The internet is the public's main source of diet and nutrition information, and seeking health-related information is one of the most common reasons for searching the internet (Jones and Fox 2009; Cash et al. 2015; Ofcom 2018). Moreover, research suggests that people are also tracking and sharing their diet, weight, and exercise routines via social media, blogs, and fitness apps (Fox 2011). This can be to keep track of calorie, nutrient, and activity intake via smartphone applications such as MyFitnessPal, which also has a social media platform where users can share their activity and progress with other users. This ability to engage with nutrition information online is important given that an unhealthy diet is linked to a range of non-communicable diseases such as stroke and is a contributing factor in around 20% of global deaths (The Lancet Global Health 2018). Thus, having access to good nutrition information online arguably can have many benefits, such as informing pro-health behaviours (Cousineau et al. 2008; Cugelman et al. 2011; Pollard et al. 2015).

However, whilst there are many documented benefits of having access to nutrition and health information, concern has been raised over the level of misinformation available to consumers online (Eysenbach and Powell 2002; Wansink 2006; Hausenblas 2015; Ramondt and Ramírez 2019). The level of concern is partly a reflection of the fact that people can model their eating habits based on what they are seeing online (Cruwys et al. 2015; Higgs 2015). Higgs (2015) argues that we may choose to model the eating behaviour of others due to motivations to be part of a group and to feel liked/accepted. Another reason proposed by Higgs states that people model eating behaviour for informational purposes (knowing what constitutes 'correct' eating behaviour). Here, people seek guidance from others to fill an information void and to increase self-efficacy, and they model behaviour they see because they want to reduce the uncertainty they feel (Morahan-Martin 2004; Cruwys et al. 2015). Further, Lambert and colleagues (2019) found that participants did not follow official dietary guidelines because there is no sense of urgency; focusing on long-term reduction of risk factors is something that their participants would worry about later in life. Instead, participants were likely to follow what they see on social media because they want a particular body image (see also Chapter 4). Females, in particular, were prone to thinking that if they wanted to look like people they see on social media and in advertisements then they need to eat like those on social media. Further still, there is evidence to suggest that people are more likely to follow the eating norms of a group if they find that group aspirational (Cruwys et al. 2015). There is also limited research to suggest that a range of moderating factors may influence whether someone models the behaviour of others, including age (young), weight (overweight), personality (impulsive), and (low) self-esteem; these moderating factors are strongest when looking at the interaction between participant and model (e.g., eating behaviour is likely to be modelled if participant and model are of similar age or weight; Bevelander et al. 2013; Cruwys et al. 2015).

Fad diets and social media trends

Two interrelated ways that NM can flourish online and reach so many people is through social media trends and the promotion of fad diets.

The convincing presentation of the fad diet

Fad diets such as low-carb/high fat diets (LCHF, e.g., the Atkins Diet), the Paleo diet, the Cabbage Soup Diet, and the Raw Food Diet typically promise speedy weight loss results, involve eating a restrictive diet that bans certain foods, may involve the addition of certain 'magical' fat-burning foods, or involve taking large quantities of supplements (Porter 2017). Whilst some of these diets have more support than others from the scientific literature (for instance the LCHF diet, Foster et al. 2003), all lack sufficient scientific backing in terms of their effects on various health markers (e.g., weight) over longer periods of time (Kuchkuntla et al. 2018). Further, all fad diets promote NM in the sense that they contradict established and official dietary guidelines; they are ineffective, heavily restrict people's eating habits, or simply are not sufficiently supported by scientific research (Foster et al. 2003; Kuchkuntla et al. 2018). Proponents of various diets have also been accused of sensationalising and making unsubstantiated claims about a diet, food, or supplement (Rousseau 2015). For example, Tim Ferriss, who is a popular and influential American author, blogger, and entrepreneur, publishes podcasts on a variety of topics relating to health and self-improvement. In 2015, Ferriss aired a podcast with Dr D'Agostino,

Associate Professor in Molecular Pharmacology and Physiology. The podcast was titled *Dom D'Agostino on Fasting, Ketosis, and the End of Cancer* (Ferriss 2015). In this podcast, Ferris and Dr D'Agostino discuss how a ketogenic diet can be used to kill cancer cells. The title of the podcast is clearly misleading, and the podcast presents a one-sided and overly simplistic view of the very complex topic of linking diet to cancer treatment. Indeed, in follow-up interviews, Dr D'Agostino apparently conceded that the title of the podcast is 'unfortunate' and that, whilst a ketogenic diet can kill or slow down the growth of some cancer cells, it can speed up others (Easter 2019).

Even if the evidence were to support the benefits of an LCHF diet for all outcomes (i.e., not just weight loss, but other health indicators such as blood pressure and insulin resistance), the way that this diet is promoted online is often filled with misinformation and unhealthy advice (Mann et al. 2014; Holmberg 2015). For example, an internet search for the ketogenic diet (an LCHF diet) brings up many images of processed meats, which are not exactly healthy; in fact, processed meats have been declared carcinogenic by the World Health Organisation (Bouvard et al. 2015). Similarly, popular versions of the LCHF diet such as the Atkins Diet discourages the consumption of many fruits, vegetables, and wholegrains, which contradicts most official nutrition guidelines and many current studies relating to fibre consumption, gut health, and health outcomes (Dahl and Stewart 2015). Thus, whilst the LCHF might achieve weight loss and can be adopted relatively healthily, the messages that are often communicated in the promotion of such diets can be misleading, contradictory, and unhealthy.

One of the reasons the fad diet is able to flourish online is that communicators generally provide an overly simplistic argument and refuse to include a full and accountable discussion of the scientific evidence, which is often contradictory and changes frequently. Rousseau (2015) gives the example of comedian Dara O'Briain in 2009 saying that one way to spot pseudoscience is that it claims certainty where none exists and that science, on the other hand, 'knows it doesn't know everything. Otherwise it would stop' (O'Briain 2009). Further, fad diets also often fail to stipulate the objectives or desired outcomes of those diets, which can add to the confusion of deciding whether a particular diet is right for you. Indeed, 'Eating well' means different things, depending on the approach you take. For example, whether our priority is the environment, animal welfare, body fat, blood glucose levels, inflammatory markers, agriculture, or general physical health will all determine what it means to eat well. That is, eating well will mean different things in each of these contexts (Jackson 2017).

The complexity of nutrition science-based evidence and the attractive simplicity of the messages provided by many of the non-experts offering advice online has meant that a misleading, overly simplified message that is not backed up by evidence, but by testimonials and often endorsed by celebrities, is becoming the new trusted source for those looking for quick and effective solutions to their health and weight-related problems (Ayoob et al. 2002; Rousseau 2015). This situation, where essentially anyone can dish out nutrition advice and can do it in a more accessible or convincing way than scientists or official sources of information, is leading to a crisis of authority (Wansink 2006; Belasco 2013; Holmberg 2015). Specifically, when online sources of information can make themselves seem credible, generate a coherent and focused argument, and use motivating examples as evidence, consumers (at least some of them) are led to question the legitimacy of official sources of nutrition information, which are often contradictory (Holmberg 2015; Rousseau 2015).

#Trends

In addition to the online promotion of specific diets that are potentially harmful to consumers, online platforms like social media encourage the formation of lifestyle trends. By way of example, *#thinspiration* (a combination of the words thin and inspiration) and *#fitspiration* on social media platforms such as Instagram, Twitter, and Facebook are two main trends that are discussed here in order to demonstrate how nutrition misinformation can flourish and how it can be harmful. Indeed, one mechanism through which nutrition misinformation can spread rapidly to large audiences is through the hashtag (#)—a convenient and organised way for people to read about topics that follow a specific theme. Further, social media and websites make it easier for trends to form because they create a situation where people can easily seek information that confirms already held beliefs. This can be a strong facilitator of trends, where one can not only find information that acts as confirmation of one's opinions, but one can also seek other people to interact with in real-time who share those same beliefs, thus reinforcing those beliefs even further (Wansink et al. 2014).

All the trends discussed here have implications for the nutritional knowledge and behaviours of the public, with some communicating extremely harmful information. Furthermore, they have in common the fact that they typically involve people posting pictures of themselves and sharing information about their daily eating and exercise habits in order to inspire others. For example, *#thinspiration* (which is closely associated with the pro-anorexia movement) promotes pro-anorexic beliefs and behaviours, and heavily suggests that eating disorders are not an illness but rather a lifestyle choice (Fox et al. 2005; Boero and Pascoe 2012; Crowe and Watts 2016; Talbot et al. 2017). Worryingly, a quick Twitter search of *#thinspiration* brings up many tweets from people, mainly young women, posting pictures of themselves in order to inspire others to aim for a level of thinness that can only realistically be achieved by adopting behaviours associated with eating disorders (Fox et al. 2005). Some give tips on how to suppress hunger, such as taking up smoking, followed by hashtags such as *#ihatemyself*. Further, searching Instagram for the term *thinspo* also brings up many worrying posts related to diet and lifestyle choices, where people share their extreme diets (often involving very little food or encouraging purging after eating) and seek encouragement for their behaviour.

Similarly, *#fitspiration* is a current social media trend that promotes images of individuals who look exceedingly fit, with toned, muscular bodies. The idea is to inspire people to maintain a healthy lifestyle, with a significant focus on physical activity and eating to achieve and maintain an athletic body (Hausenblas 2015). There is research to suggest that the fitspiration trend promotes more positive images and a healthier lifestyle than its thinspiration counterpart (Talbot et al. 2017). This is due in part because one presumably needs to actually eat some food and engage in physical activity to achieve the type of fit/athletic image that is being celebrated. There is also some evidence to suggest that fitspiration is also more popular than thinspiration (Simpson and Mazzeo 2017). However, research has demonstrated that despite claiming that health and fitness is the goal being projected in fitspiration posts, it is actually attractiveness, and subsequently thinness, that is the primary objective (Simpson and Mazzeo 2017). Indeed, it just takes a quick search for 'fitspiration' on social media sites like Pinterest and Instagram and you will be confronted with images of extremely and sometimes worryingly thin women. Of course, all of this gives the impression that one should exercise and eat to maintain a desirable appearance rather than to maintain one's physical and mental health (Carrotte et al. 2017). As a result, nutrition misinformation is rife in these environments, with many unqualified people sharing diet advice, based on the latest fad diets (Villiard and Moreno 2012). Similarly, pro-muscularity websites, blogs, and forums provide an intense focus on building muscular bodies and offer dietary guidelines to achieve them (Murray et al. 2016). Like fitspiration, the communication of bodybuilding information initially seems relatively healthy. However, research suggests that the content of pro-muscularity websites displays characteristics and behaviours that are very similar to the characteristics of eating disorders; for example, periods of highly restrictive eating with periods of bingeing on a lot of food, which is often unhealthy (Mosley 2009; Murray et al. 2012, 2013, 2016).

The culprits: sharers of nutrition misinformation online

The sharers of NM online are varied, ranging from people who are deliberately sharing misinformation in an attempt to gain publicity and economic/professional gain (e.g., Belle Gibson, discussed previously) to regular consumers of information who either share it because they believe the information is true or who share it because they think others will find it interesting (Chen et al. 2015). The next section highlights some of the most common types of sharers of NM.

The health and fitness industry and the rise of the micro-celebrity

In the nutrition and fitness sector, there is a proliferation of entrepreneurs and personalities using the online environment to market products and services. Indeed, industry plays a significant role in the growth of the online marketing of nutrition information, as food and supplement companies adopt a wide range of social media strategies to promote their products to consumers (Belz and Schmidt-Riediger 2010; Holmberg 2016). For example, whilst they engage in direct marketing campaigns on social media (Strom 2011), companies can also distance themselves from their own marketing campaigns by employing or sponsoring individuals to advertise their products online. For instance, Optimum Nutrition, a popular supplement company offering a range of protein, sport, and health supplements, sponsor 'athletes' to promote their products. These sponsored athletes, according to the Optimum Nutrition website, have a range of different professions, including bodybuilding, modelling, and 'influencer'—the latter having a rather ambiguous relationship to the word athlete. Typically, the sponsored 'athletes' for supplement companies and food brands already have an established social media following and are paid to continue their usual social media activities while occasionally promoting the product they are being paid to promote.

Celebrities and healthy-living bloggers, too, are paid by supplement and food companies to advertise products online. Typically, healthy-living bloggers maintain an internet presence as a way to document and share their daily activities and behaviours, in the hope of inspiring or showing others how to live a similar lifestyle (Boepple and Thompson 2014). Social media influencers who have more than 100,000 followers can be paid up to £4,000 for a single post that advertises a product or company, while this can rise to £230,000 for a YouTube video if the person has 7 million followers or more (O'Connor 2017).

The advancement of Web 2.0 and this culture of paying people for having a large social media following has resulted in the rise of the micro-celebrity (i.e., people who become famous because of their social media presence). Certainly, there is a documented rise in self-branding, where individuals can develop a distinctive public image in the hope of attracting financial, professional, or social capital gain (Khamis et al. 2017). In this environment, it is easy to see how misinformation, and by extent, harmful advertising, can proliferate. Indeed, there are many recent examples where personalities have been attracting attention from the Advertising Standards Authority (ASA) for providing misleading advertisements, and those being investigated are only the tip of the iceberg (Tait 2019). One example is provided by a reality TV star posting a photo of herself on Instagram looking like she is about to eat a burger and fries. The photo was accompanied by the text: 'Always take my @ProteinWorld[2] Carb Blockers Before a Cheat meal, contain natural ingredients and stop any unused sugars being used as fat #ad' (Calvert 2018). The ASA ruled that the advert—and others like it posted by other celebrities around the same time—was misleading and gave the impression that consumers could eat high carb foods and not worry about storing fat.

It is not just micro-celebrities and reality TV stars who attract criticism for their endorsement of diets and nutrition products. For example, Hollywood actress turned wellness guru Gwyneth Paltrow has developed a lifestyle brand, *Goop*. Through this brand, Paltrow has attracted criticism for promoting highly restrictive diets, as the following quote indicates: 'I see patients suffering with anorexia nervosa and now I'm reading their diet in pamphlet form'. This is a statement made by Catherine Collins, a dietician at St George's hospital, London (cited in Wilcox 2011). The concern is in reference to a diet that severely restricts the number of foods one can eat and results in dieters exercising for around two hours per day whilst often eating fewer than 700 calories per day (Wilcox 2011). According to Wilcox, who tried the diet and documented the process, the first week of the diet recommends that dieters eat only seven different foods (mostly vegetables, with a little protein), and most of this should be blended. Having reviewed the diet that Wilcox is following, Collins says, 'The lack of absorbable calcium means you risk early onset osteoporosis and osteopenia—something that Gwyneth Paltrow has been diagnosed with'.

Harm caused by nutrition misinformation

This section addresses some of main potential outcomes consumers are faced with when regularly exposed to fraud and misinformation of this nature.

Psychological harm

The psychological harms which may be incurred from NM can cause negative emotions amongst users. Indeed, psychological consequences from NM may also result in a distorted view of body image (Croll 2005). When consumers are constantly shown images of models who are of a specific body image (e.g., 'positively' thin, or 'negatively' large), they are prone to experience a sense of peer pressure to abide by these standards (Dunkley et al. 2001). Hence, this leads them to adhere to specific diets and possibly experience feelings of intense discontent towards their own body image if the misinformation causes opposite effects to happen. Indeed, there is a growing body of research that suggests that social media trends such as fitspiration and thinspiration can affect mood, self-esteem, and body dissatisfaction (Tiggemann and Zaccardo 2015; Holland and Tiggemann 2016; Prichard et al. 2018). Of course, the outcome of this can lead to eating disturbances; these include, but are not limited to, anorexia and bulimia nervosa (Juarex et al. 2012; Saunders and Eaton 2018).

Further, there is evidence to suggest that the prevalence of trends such as raw food diets, clean eating, and the promotion of food fear have resulted in dramatic increases of orthorexia nervosa (ON), which received proposals for specific diagnostic criteria in 2015 for the first time (Santarossa et al. 2019). ON refers to disordered eating behaviour generated by a compulsive obsession for biologically pure and healthy nutrition (Moroze et al. 2015), going as far as avoiding food that has been sliced/prepared a certain way or foods that have any 'undesirable' components, such as fat or sugar. Those suffering from ON often face extreme dietary restrictions, social isolation, and malnutrition (Moroze et al. 2015).

In addition, unnecessary feelings of guilt and self-blame may be present in cases where one does not abide to the food misinformation diet which are assumed to be correct (Khawandah and Tewfik 2016). In many cases, diets are unsustainable, and individuals who are unable to lose weight in a short amount of time may feel resentment and anger towards their bodies (Raggat et al. 2018). This can result in social isolation from peers due to frustration and mood swings from feeling dissatisfied with one's body image (Smith-Jackson et al. 2011). Those who are regularly exposed to this type of information may feel inadequate in their perceived ability to confidently manage a healthy lifestyle, thus being more susceptible to following misinformation (Ayoob et al. 2002). In addition, consumers of frequent misinformation may fall into depression upon finding out that they were being scammed and their health goals were not met (Khawandah and Tewfik 2016).

Physical harm

Physical harm which may occur from NM can include deterioration in health and sickness. For instance, there may be toxic components in foods or supplements which can cause severe sickness and adverse reactions to the body, such as sports mixtures that cause gastrointestinal discomfort (Brouns et al. 2002). This situation has been exacerbated by the online environment, which also enables people to purchase products that are not legally sold in the consumer's country of origin (e.g., slimming pills not approved for sale in a consumer's country). This unregulated trade has led to significant physical harm to the consumer, with a fatality being a possible outcome. One such example is the death of Eloise Parry, a 21-year-old British student who suffered from bulimia. Eloise bought diet pills online and became addicted to the chemical components of the pills. Three people from London went on trial for manslaughter after buying chemicals from China and manufacturing the pills in their London flat (*BBC* 2018).

Further, for the average consumer as well as athletes, there are clear health implications for the copious amounts of supplement products that are marketed towards those wishing to improve their physical performance, their body, and their general physical and mental health. Indeed, many of the online-marketed products contain ingredients that could be considered unhealthy. For example, large amounts of artificial flavours and sweeteners and many heavy metal contaminants such as lead, arsenic, and mercury are a known problem in supplements (Ernst 2002; Saper et al. 2008).

In addition, NM can cause the development of unhealthy eating habits and diet (Harrison 2005), which has direct implications for physical health. For example, NM may result in a number of serious weight issues, including the possibility to fall into levels of obesity, which can lead to heart attack, liver failure, and mobility issues (Harrison 2005; Raggatt et al. 2018). On the other hand, rapid weight loss may also occur due to the lack of nutrients (Khawandah and Tewfik 2016). In addition, the 'yo-yo' effect (weight loss and weight gain in a short time) may lead to cardiovascular disease, renal dysfunction, and osteoporosis (Khawandah and Tewfik 2016). Taken together, these weight issues may lead to a decreased quality of life, with an increase in early mortality.

Economic harm

The main economic harm from nutrition misinformation comes from unnecessary financial expenditure by consumers, who pay for ineffective or unnecessary diet and health products (British Nutrition Foundation 2015; Manning and Soon 2016). This may be particularly problematic for those from a lower socio-economic background, leading to serious financial turmoil. For example, trends such as gluten-free, organic, and dairy-free require the purchasing of alternative products that are more expensive; thus it has been advised by the British Dietetic Association that any diet promoting those expensive food alternatives should only be followed if there is a diagnosed medical reason to do so (Porter 2017).

A further example of the economic cost of the promotion of various misinformation in supplements comes from the fact that protein powders are now painted as a necessity for anyone wishing to gain muscle and lose fat. There are many examples of people who are sponsored by supplement companies suggesting that it is imperative to consume a protein shake immediately after your workout. For example, Shaun Stafford, who is an Optimum Nutrition–sponsored athlete, is frequently posting on Instagram about how imperative it is to take a quality protein supplement. When doing a question-and-answer session on Instagram in October 2018, Shaun was asked how he recovers from workouts, to which he responded,

> When it comes to recovery, it is *really* important for your diet to be on point. This means not only the food you are eating, but also the sports nutrition you are using. So, for me, Gold Standard Whey is a key part of that.

Further discussion and conclusion: from misinformed to informed

A central component of the argument set out in this chapter is that NM has been able to flourish in the online environment because evidence-based nutrition evidence is complex and difficult to understand by the public (Goldberg and Sliwa 2011). This, along with the accessibility of Web 2.0, has created an opportunity for many different voices to communicate nutrition information to large audiences. Many of these voices are unqualified, presenting erroneous, biased, or fraudulent information to consumers. This is problematic because NM is associated with psychological, physical, and economic harms. The number of conflicting, sometimes erroneous, and often convincing messages that consumers are exposed to has led to concern over whether consumers are experiencing information overload, which may result in people making poor nutrition decisions (Ramondt and Ramírez 2019).

In addition to encouraging fact checking by consumers (Chen et al. 2015), those who communicate NM should be encouraged to provide a more balanced and measured representation of the nutrition evidence. One way to do this is through the regulation of the way industry and individuals advertise products and services, both online and offline (Nestle 2013; Tempels et al. 2017; Leon and Ken 2019).

Ensuring adverts are not misleading or harmful currently falls under the remit of the ASA in the United Kingdom and, whilst they have been active in investigating complaints against those communicating misinformation, they have been able to have only a minimal impact (Tait 2019). It is not only in relation to advertisements that regulation could be improved. As indicated, there is an observed problem of weight loss and nutrition supplements either containing harmful ingredients or containing such poor-quality ingredients that they are ineffective. Therefore, in order for the nutrition information environment to be safe, there needs to be fundamental changes in the way that food and supplements are produced and marketed.

Addressing the problem of how NM is instantaneously communicated online to many people is imperative given that social influence, eating norms, and personal factors such as self-esteem all play a significant role in determining what people eat (Bevelander et al. 2013; Higgs 2015). Because of this, it is vital for there to be more positive and healthy role models accessible online and capable of engaging with audiences to the same extent as their less healthy counterparts. Luckily, some qualified medical and dietitian professionals have developed a substantial online presence and are using their influence to improve health: *The Doctor's Kitchen* and the *Gut Health Doctor* are two examples this. This is important because if there are more qualified professionals who can generate a significant social presence—and can communicate accurate and healthy messages to their audience—then this might work to reduce the crisis of legitimacy experienced by official sources of nutrition information (Holmberg 2015; Rousseau 2015). It may also help to reduce the psychological, physical, and economic harms association with nutrition misinformation.

Notes

1 For information on the training programme, see www.bodybuilding.com/workout-plans/kris-gethins-8-week-hardcore-video-trainer.

2 The @ symbol preceding the target word, in this case ProteinWorld, gives the user a direct link to the company.

References

Ashley JM and Jarvis WT (1995) Position of the American dietetic association, *Journal of the American Dietetic Association* 95(6):705–707

Ayoob KT, Duyff RL and Quagliani D (2002) Position of the American dietetic association: food and nutrition misinformation, *Journal of the American Dietetic Association* 102(2):260–266

BBC (2018) Eloise Parry: Diet pills caused 'distressing death'. Available at: www.bbc.co.uk/news/uk-england-shropshire-44127048

Belz FM and Schmidt-Riediger B (2010) Marketing strategies in the age of sustainable development: evidence from the food industry. *Business Strategy and the Environment* 19(7):401–416

Bevelander KE, Anschütz DJ, Creemers DHM, Kleinjan M, Engels RCME (2013) The role of explicit and implicit self-esteem in peer modeling of palatable food intake: a study on social media interaction among youngsters'. *PLoS One* 8(8):e72481

Boepple L and Thompson JK (2014) A content analysis of healthy living blogs: evidence of content thematically consistent with dysfunctional eating attitudes and behaviors. *International Journal of Eating Disorders* 47(4):362–367

Boero N and Pascoe CJ (2012) Pro-anorexia communities and online interaction: bringing the pro-ana body online. *Body and Society* 18(2):27–57

Bouvard V, Loomis D, Guyton KZ, Grosse Y, El Ghissassi F, Benbrahim-Tallaa L, Guha N, Mattock H and Straif K (2015) Carcinogenicity of consumption of red and processed meat. *The Lancet Oncology* 16(16):1599–1600

British Nutrition Foundation (2015) *Nutrition for sport and exercise*. Available at: www.nutrition.org.uk/healthyliving/an-active-lifestyle/eating-for-sport-and-exercise.html?showall=1&limitstart=

Brouns F, Nieuwenhoven Mv, Jeukendrup A and Lichtenbelt M (2002) Functional foods and food supplements for athletes: from myths to benefit claims substantiation through the study of selected biomarkers. *British Journal of Nutrition* 88(S2):177–186

Calvert W (2018) Holly Hagan's plug for Protein World pills banned by advertising watchdog for making misleading health claims. *The Sun*. Available at: www.thesun.co.uk/money/5857784/holly-hagens-protein-world-ad-banned-by-advertising-watchdog-for-making-misleading-health-claims/

Carrotte ER, Prichard I and Lim MSC (2017) Fitspiration on social media: a content analysis of gendered images. *Journal of Medical Internet Research* 19(3):e95

Cash T, Desbrow B, Leveritt M and Ball L (2015) Utilization and preference of nutrition information sources in Australia. *Health Expectations* 18(6):2288–2295

Chen X, Sin SCJ, Theng Y and Lee CS (2015) Why students share misinformation on social media: motivation, gender, and study-level differences. *Journal of Academic Librarianship* 41(5):583–592

Cousineau T, Houle B, Bromberg J, Fernandez KC and Kling WC (2008) A pilot study of an online workplace nutrition program: the value of participant input in program development. *Journal of Nutrition Education and Behavior* 40(3):160–167

Croll J (2005) Body image and adolescents. In J Stang J and Story M (eds.) Guidelines for adolescent nutrition services. Minneapolis: University of Minnesota

Crowe N and Watts M (2016) 'We're just like Gok, but in reverse': Ana Girls – empowerment and resistance in digital communities. *International Journal of Adolescence and Youth* 21(3):379–390

Cruwys T, Bevelander KE and Hermans RCJ (2015) Social modeling of eating: a review of when and why social influence affects food intake and choice. *Appetite* 86:3–18

Cugelman B, Thelwall M and Dawes P (2011) Online interventions for social marketing health behavior change campaigns: a meta-analysis of psychological architectures and adherence factors. *Journal of Medical Internet Research* 13(1):1–17

Dahl WJ and Stewart ML (2015) Position of the academy of nutrition and dietetics: health implications of dietary fiber. *Journal of the Academy of Nutrition and Dietetics* 115(11):1861–1870

Davey M (2015) Jessica Ainscough, Australia's 'wellness warrior', dies of cancer aged 30. *The Guardian*. Available at: www.theguardian.com/australia-news/2015/mar/01/jessica-ainscough-australia-wellness-warrior-dies-cancer-aged-30

Easter M (2019) Keto Diet history: how the ketogenic diet went mainstream. *Men's Health*. Available at: www.menshealth.com/nutrition/a25775330/keto-diet-history/

Ernst E (2002) Adulteration of Chinese herbal medicines with synthetic drugs: a systematic review. *Journal of Internal Medicine* 252(2):107–113

Eysenbach G and Powell J (2002) Empirical studies assessing the quality of health information for consumers: a systematic review. *Journal of the American Medical Association* 287(20):2691–2700

Ferriss T (2015) Dom D'Agostino on fasting, ketosis, and the end of cancer. *The Tim Ferriss Show*. Available at: https://tim blog/2015/11/03/dominic-dagostino/

Foster GD, Wyatt HR, Hill JO, McGuckin BG, Brill C, Mohammed BS, Szapary PO, Rader DJ, Edman JS and Klein S (2003) A randomized trial of a low-carbohydrate diet for obesity. *New England Journal of Medicine* 348(21):2082–2090

Fox NJ, Ward KJ and O'Rourke AJO (2005) Pro-anorexia, weight-loss drugs and the internet: an 'anti-recovery' explanatory model of anorexia. *Sociology of Health & Illness* 27:944–971

Fox S (2011) *The social life of health information, pew internet and American life project*. Available at: www.pewinternet.org/2011/05/12/the-social-life-of-health-information-2011/

Gerson C and Walker M (2001) *The Gerson therapy: the proven nutritional program for cancer and other illnesses*. New York: Kensington Publishing

Goldberg JP and Sliwa SA (2011) Communicating actionable nutrition messages: challenges and opportunities. *Proceedings of the Nutrition Society* 70(1):26–37

Harrison K (2005). Is 'fat free' good for me? A panel study of television viewing and children's nutritional knowledge and reasoning. *Health Communication* 17(2):117–132

Hausenblas H (2015) Is 'fitspiration' doing more harm than good? | Eat + Run | *US News*. Available at: https://health.usnews.com/health-news/blogs/eat-run/2015/02/09/is-fitspiration-doing-more-harm-than-good?int=9fe908%26src=usn_fb

Higgs S (2015) Social norms and their influence on eating behaviours. *Appetite* 86:38–4

Holland G and Tiggemann M (2016) A systematic review of the impact of the use of social networking sites on body image and disordered eating outcomes. *Body Image* 17:100–110

Holmberg C (2015) Politicization of the low-carb high-fat diet in Sweden, promoted on social media by non-conventional experts. *International Journal of E-Politics* 6(3)

Holmberg C (2016) If you can't beat it-use it: why and how clinicians need to consider social media in the treatment of adolescents with obesity. *European Journal of Clinical Nutrition* 70(9):977–978

Jackson P (2017) Eating well. *Geoforum* 84:239–240

Jones S and Fox S (2009) *Pew internet project data demo: generations online in 2009, pew internet and American life project*. Available at: www.pewinternet.org/2009/01/28/generations-online-in-2009/

Juarez L, Soto E and Pritchard ME (2012) Drive for muscularity and drive for thinness: the impact of pro-anorexia websites. *Eating Disorders* 20(2):99–112

Khamis S, Ang L and Welling R (2017) Self-branding, 'micro-celebrity' and the rise of social media influencers. *Celebrity Studies* 8(2):191–208

Khawandanah J and Tewfik I (2016) Fad diets: lifestyle promises and health challenges. *Journal of Food Research* 5(6):80–94

Krumbeck JA, Maldonado-Gomez MX, Ramer-Tail AE and Hutkins RW (2016) Prebiotics and synbiotics: dietary strategies for improving gut health. *Current Opinion in Gastroenterology* 32(2):110–119

Kuchkuntla AR, Limketkai B, Narda S, Hurt RT and Mundi MS (2018) Fad diets: hype or hope? *Current Nutrition Reports* 7(4):310–323

Lambert M, Chivers P and Farringdon F (2019) In their own words: a qualitative study exploring influences on the food choices of university students. *Health Promotion Journal of Australia* 30(1):66–75

Lavorgna A and Sugiura L (2018) Caught in a lie: the rise and fall of a respectable deviant. *Deviant Behavior* (online first)

Leon KS and Ken I (2019) Legitimized fraud and the state-corporate criminology of food: a spectrum-based theory. *Crime, Law and Social Change* 71(1):25–46

Ma T and Atkin D (2017) User generated content and credibility evaluation of online health information: a meta analytic study. *Telematics and Informatics* 34(5):472–486

Mann J, McLean R, Skeaff M and Morenga LT (2014) Low carbohydrate diets: going against the grain. *The Lancet* 384(9953):1479–1480

Manning L and Soon JM (2016) Food safety, food fraud, and food defense: a fast evolving literature. *Journal of Food Science* 81(4):R823–R834

Morahan-Martin JM (2004) How internet users find, evaluate, and use online health information: a cross-cultural review. *CyberPsychology & Behavior* 7(5):497–510

Moroze RM, Dunn TM, Holland C, Yager J and Waintraub P (2015) Microthinking about micronutrients: a case of transition from obsessions about healthy eating to near-fatal 'orthorexia nervosa' and proposed diagnostic criteria. *Psychosomatics* 56(4):397–403

Mosley PE (2009) Bigorexia: bodybuilding and muscle dysmorphia. *European Eating Disorders Review* 17(3):191–198

Murray SB, Griffiths S, Hazery L, Shen T, Wooldridge T and Mond JM (2016) Go big or go home: a thematic content analysis of pro-muscularity websites. *Body Image* 16:17–20

Murray SB, Griffiths S, Rieger E and Touyz SW (2013) A comparison of compulsive exercise in male and female presentations of anorexia nervosa: what is the difference? *Advances in Eating Disorders: Theory, Research & Practice* 2(1):65–70

Murray SB, Rieger E, Hildebrandt T, Karlov L, Russell J, Boon E, Dawson RT and Touyz SW (2012) A comparison of eating, exercise, shape, and weight related symptomatology in males with muscle dysmorphia and anorexia nervosa. *Body Image* 9(2):193–200

Nestle M (2013) *Food politics: how the food industry influences nutrition and health. Revised tenth anniversary expanded edition*. Oakland, CA: University of California Press

O'Briain D (2009) Science doesn't know everything. Available at: www.youtube.com/watch?v=uDYba0m6ztE

O'Connor C (2017) Earning power: how much money can top influencers bank per post? *Forbes*. Available at: www.forbes.com/sites/clareoconnor/2017/06/20/earning-power-how-much-money-can-top-influencers-bank-per-post/#47aef0c2a6e4

Ofcom (2018) *Adults' media use and attitudes report*. London: Office of Communications

Phillip A (2015) 'None of it's true': Disgraced wellness guru Belle Gibson comes clean on cancer hoax. *The Washington Post*. Available at: https://www.washingtonpost.com/news/to-your-health/wp/2015/04/22/none-of-its-true-disgraced-wellness-guru-belle-gibson-comes-clean-on-cancer-hoax/

Pollard CM, Pulker CE, Meng X, Kerr DA and Scott JA (2015) Who uses the internet as a source of nutrition and dietary information? an Australian population perspective. *Journal of Medical Internet Research* 17(8):1–14

Porter S (2017) *Food fact sheet: fad diets*. British Dietetic Association. Available at: www.bda.uk.com/foodfacts

Prichard I, McLachlan AC, Lavis T and Tiggemann M (2018) The impact of different forms of #fitspiration imagery on body image, mood, and self-objectification among young women. *Sex Roles* 78(11–12):789–798

Public Health England (2016) *The eatwell guide*. Available at: www.gov.uk/government/publications/the-eatwell-guide

Raggatt M, Wright CJ, Carrotte E, Jenkinson R, Mulgrew K, Prichard I and Lim MS (2018) 'I aspire to look and feel healthy like the posts convey': engagement with fitness inspiration on social media and perceptions of its influence on health and wellbeing. *BMC Public Health* 18(1):1002

Ramondt S and Ramírez AS (2019) Assessing the impact of the public nutrition information environment: adapting the cancer information overload scale to measure diet information overload. *Patient Education and Counseling* 102(1):37–42

Rousseau S (2015) The celebrity quick-fix: when good food meets bad science. *Food, Culture and Society* 18(2):265–287

Rudd M and House L (2018) No makeup, body hair and a coconut bra: why controversial vegan blogger Freelee the Banana Girl fled the city to lead an off-grid life in the JUNGLE – and you won't believe how much money she's saved. *Daily Mail Online.* Available at: www.dailymail.co.uk/femail/article-5872459/Why-vegan-blogger-Freelee-Banana-Girl-fled-city-live-grid-life-forest.html

Santarossa S, Lacasse J, Larocque J and Woodruff SJ (2019) #Orthorexia on Instagram: a descriptive study exploring the online conversation and community using the Netlytic software. *Eating and Weight Disorders* 24(2):283–290

Saper RB, Phillips RS, Sehgal A, Khouri N, Davis RB, Paquin J, Thuppil V and Kales SN (2008) Lead, mercury, and arsenic in US- and Indian-manufactured Ayurvedic medicines sold via the internet. *JAMA – Journal of the American Medical Association* 300(8):915–923

Saunders JF and Eaton AA (2018) Snaps, selfies, and shares: how three popular social media platforms contribute to the sociocultural model of disordered eating among young women. *Cyberpsychology, Behavior, and Social Networking* 21(6):343–354

Simpson CC and Mazzeo SE (2017) Skinny is not enough: a content analysis of fitspiration on Pinterest. *Health Communication* 32(5):560–567

Smith-Jackson T, Reel JJ and Thackeray R (2011) Coping with 'bad body image days': strategies from first-year young adult college women. *Body Image* 8(4):335–342

Strom S (2011) Pepsi contest faces more charges of cheating. *The New York Times.* Available at: www.nytimes.com/2011/01/06/business/06charity.html

Tait A (2019) Forcing social-media influencers to be clear about #ads? Good luck with that. *The Guardian.* Available at: www.theguardian.com/commentisfree/2019/jan/25/social-media-influencers-clear-ads-celebrities-authorities

Talbot CV, Gavin J, van Steen T and Morey Y (2017) A content analysis of thinspiration, fitspiration, and bonespiration imagery on social media. *Journal of Eating Disorders* 5(40)

Tempels T, Verweij M and Blok V (2017) Big food's ambivalence: seeking profit and responsibility for health. *American Journal of Public Health* 107(3):402–406

The Lancet Global Health (2018) Getting to the heart of non-communicable diseases. Editorial. *The Lancet Global Health* 6(9):e933

Tiggemann M and Zaccardo M (2015) 'Exercise to be fit, not skinny': the effect of fitspiration imagery on women's body image. *Body Image* 15:61–67

Ventola CL (2014) Social media and health care professionals: benefits, risks, and best practices. *P & T: A Peer-Reviewed Journal for Formulary Management* 39(7):491–520

Villiard H and Moreno MA (2012) Fitness on Facebook: advertisements generated in response to profile content. *Cyberpsychology, Behavior, and Social Networking* 15(10):564–568

Wansink B (2006) Position of the American dietetic association: food and nutrition misinformation. *Journal of the American Dietetic Association* 106(4):601–607

Wansink B, Tal A and Brumberg A (2014) Ingredient-based food fears and avoidance: antecedents and antidotes. *Food Quality and Preference* 38:40–48

Wilcox, R. (2011) Gwyneth Paltrow's personal trainer Tracy Anderson's diet plan gave me blackouts. *Daily Mail.* Available at: https://www.dailymail.co.uk/health/article-1367879/Gwyneth-Paltrows-personal-trainer-Tracy-Andersons-diet-plan-gave-blackouts.html

Winter K (2014) 'I eat 51 bananas a day!' Self-proclaimed 'diet guru' says her toned physique is down to the MOUNTAINS of fruit she eats. *Daily Mail.* Available at: www.dailymail.co.uk/femail/article-2601633/I-eat-51-bananas-day-Self-proclaimed-diet-guru-claims-toned-physique-MOUNTAINS-fruit-eats-single-meal-time.html

9 Activism against medicine on social media

Untangling the #novax protest in Italy on Twitter

Anna Di Ronco and James Allen-Robertson

Introduction

Cyberspace is a rich source of health-related misinformation. Social media platforms, in particular, are used by supporters of unofficial, fraudulent, and harmful health practices and beliefs to channel potentially dangerous messages (Lavorgna and Di Ronco 2017). In the area of vaccines, pervasive misinformation on websites (Davies et al. 2002; Kata 2010) and social media (Kata 2012; Smith and Graham 2017) by anti-vaxxers (or 'no-vax' people) has been found to play a key role in shaping vaccination practices (Davies et al. 2002; Betsch et al. 2012; Kata 2012).

So far, the focus of scholarly attention has mostly been on anti-vaxxers and the content of their online messages (Kata 2010, Smith and Graham 2017), with only a few studies comparing the content of the messages of anti- and pro-vaxxers (Sak et al. 2016). Particularly missing are studies analysing the online interactions between the two groups of anti- and pro-vaxxers on social media like Twitter, which is an open digital platform with an established reputation for protest and activism (Vicari 2013). The aim of this study is to investigate whether, and to what extent, the two groups of no- and pro-vaxxers interact and engage with each other's arguments on Twitter. It does so by relying on a digital mixed method approach: (aspects of) social network analysis to detect and graphically represent Twitter communities based on their retweeting habits, measures of interaction between these communities, and virtual and visual ethnographies of Twitter posts. Research on conversations and debates on Twitter has emphasised their polarised nature (Gunnarsson Lorentzen 2014), with little interaction being established between people having different viewpoints on relevant topics (especially in terms of retweets, which usually indicate agreement and endorsement of specific statements and opinions (Ahn and Park 2015)). Even in a much-polarised debate, where different factions may not interact via retweets or even with mentions, they may still engage with the arguments of their opponents in their own tweet content. The content analysis of Twitter posts (of both their attached textual and visual material) will help investigate whether pro- and anti-vaxxers address each other's arguments in the content of their messages, in spite of their eventual limited engagement through retweets and mentions.

Critical approaches towards vaccines and vaccines-related misinformation

The debate around vaccines is much polarised with doubts on their effectiveness raised by people—generally labelled as anti-vaxxers—considered as unscientific, irrational, and contributing to health-related misinformation. As mentioned above, the public health literature on vaccines attributes to online-available anti-vaccination misinformation a considerable role in shaping vaccination practices. These practices seem to have worryingly changed and been reduced in some (especially western) countries in recent years, leading the World Health Organisation (2019) to include vaccine hesitancy among the ten threats to global health in 2019.

According to many studies (Davies et al. 2002; Betsch et al. 2012), misinformation has partly to do with the high number of internet fora appearing in online searches discussing the harms and risks of vaccines, which tend to be higher than those used by public health communicators to inform people about the perks of and need for vaccines, leaving the impression that cases where vaccines have had side effects on patients are higher in number than what they actually are. In addition, anti-vaxxers' messages also appear quite convincing and powerful in their content. These messages, indeed, often do not explicitly oppose vaccines but claim to be 'pro-safe vaccines' or to be in favour of 'vaccine choice' especially in light of the harmful substances vaccines are said to be made of (Kata 2012); in addition, anti-vaxxers' messages tend to be easy to understand and appear very credible, especially when coming from parents who use their personal stories and an emotionally-laden language to describe the negative effects they believe vaccines have caused on their children (Davies et al. 2002; Betsch et al. 2012).

Some anti-vax websites and content on social media are also more explicit and controversial than that, of course. Many speak about a conspiracy between Big Pharma and an increasingly authoritarian and totalitarian state (and the media) covering up the 'truth' about the harmfulness and ineffectiveness of vaccines to prevent infectious diseases. These ideas are often supported by way of dubious evidence (including privately published material, alternative medicine press, etc.); in addition, because of their distrust of authority, and particularly of the scientific and medical community, the offered alternative remedies tend to be 'natural' or homeopathic only (Davies et al. 2002; Kata 2010, 2012; Smith and Graham 2017). Concerned parents stumbling into these websites can of course get scared and be induced to think that immunisation practices are useless and harmful to their children and ultimately avoid them.

To address the issue of health-related misinformation, public health scholars emphasise the need to educate people (Ołpiński 2012), for instance by giving them advice on how to recognise untrustworthy online sources (Betsch et al. 2012). Other research-identified responses to misinformation include the better training of practitioners (Tafuri et al. 2014), their active use of Twitter to disseminate accurate vaccine-related information (Love et al. 2013), and the better designing of websites by health communicators (Betsch et al. 2012; Sak et al. 2016).

There is, however, another side to the debate. Critical sociologists and criminologists have emphasised the interests the pharma industry has in vaccines, as they are one of their major sources of profit (Ward 2016). In developed western countries, the interests of this industry—often intertwined with those of governments—can easily lead to an intensification of the mandatory regime around vaccines. As some have noticed, indeed, rigid immunisation regimes may be quite at odds with the NHS increased emphasis on individual's responsibility for their own health and right to informed consent (Blume 2006) and with other fundamental rights, such as the right to education (Rawlinson 2017).

By acknowledging the importance of respecting individuals' agency and rights—particularly the right to informed consent, which has much been emphasised in public health practices in recent years (Blume 2006)—and the different visions that people have on parenting, health, and attitudes towards authorities in contemporary society (Kata 2010), the literature on science and technology communication advises health communicators and institutions to engage in an open dialogue (or 'concordance', as put by Vernon 2003) with opponents. This dialogue aims (to the extent possible) at accommodating, rather than repressing or silencing, critical approaches to vaccines. Studies also highlight the importance of the public's engagement with science, including at public events (Bucchi and Trench 2014).

Study background: vaccines in Italy

Immunisation practices in Italy are regulated under the Law No. 119 of 31 July 2017, championed by Minister of Health (under the former government run by Paolo Gentiloni) Beatrice Lorenzin. This law has extended from four to ten the mandatory vaccines for children (including unaccompanied migrants) from zero to sixteen years old to protect them against polio, diphtheria, tetanus, hepatitis B, whooping cough (pertussis), haemophilus influenzae type b, measles, mumps, rubella, and chicken pox.[1] The legislative change has been justified by the government with the need to ensure herd immunity (which equals to 95% immunisation rate as recommended by the World Health Organisation), which is said to have substantially decreased in Italy both for polio (hexavalent vaccine), and measles and rubella. This has seemingly led in recent years to a 'measles outbreak', with 4,885 recorded cases and 4 deaths, following the last weekly bulletin of the Italian National Institute of Health (ISS 2017).

In the new law, provisions on mandatory vaccines are, or can be, *temporary*—they will be re-considered after three years from the entry into force of the law based on the available epidemiological data, evidence on adverse effects of vaccines, and data on vaccination coverage. The new law also introduces the administrative fine from EUR 100 to EUR 500 for parents or legal guardians who refuse to vaccinate their children, after a meeting between them and a medical practitioner who provides further information on vaccines and encourages immunisation. In addition, starting from the academic year 2019/2020, un-immunised children from zero until sixteen years old would not be able to be enrolled at school. In particular, schools have been compelled by the law to send the lists of students to the relevant local health authorities by 10 March 2018, which are to check these lists against the list of children who undertook immunisation. With the exception of the few exemptions from vaccines and the late requests for immunisation, non-vaccinated children would not be admitted at pre-school or at exams, in both primary and secondary school. The deadline of 10 March 2018 for schools to submit the list of children to the relevant local health authorities has later been postponed by the current government (see later). In addition, the process of verifying children's immunisation (which, in the original design, was to be activated by schools and carried out by the local health authority) has ultimately been replaced by a self-certification of the undergone vaccines (or scheduled appointment to undergo immunisation) by the children's parents.

Objections to this law have been raised in light of Article 32 of the Italian Constitution, the 1997 Convention on Human Rights and Biomedicine of the Council of Europe (Art. 5, 6, and 9), and the Charter of Fundamental Rights of the European Union (Art. 1 and 3)—all of which emphasise the importance of patients' informed consent in medical treatments, here seemingly obliterated by a hard-handed immunisation regime, which introduces disproportionate sanctions on children and parents. In a recent judgment instigated by the Veneto Region, the Constitutional Court (2018) has been asked to assess the legitimacy of the 10 newly introduced mandatory vaccines. According to the Court, the introduction of these 10 mandatory vaccines is justified in light of the state of the art of scientific knowledge and the available data on epidemiological safety and vaccine coverage in Italy. However, it concedes that the need for these vaccines to be mandatory may decrease in the future and lead to their reduction—at least for the four vaccines aimed at preventing measles, mumps, rubella, and chicken pox. Although the other six mandatory vaccines (against polio, diphtheria, tetanus, hepatitis B, pertussis, haemophilus influenzae type b, measles, mumps, rubella, and chicken pox) are not included in this possible revision by the law, the court suggests that 'variations in the epidemiological conditions, data on side effects and on vaccination coverage could induce the legislator to envisage a similar system that loosens the degree of coercion' also for them. In short, the Court seems to suggest that the need to reach a sufficient level of herd immunity justifies temporary mandatory governmental interventions, which are to be loosened, possibly in favour of systems that better accommodate patients' informed consent in medical treatments, once that is reached.

This new law has been antagonised by the so-called no-vax people, who have been very active on social media (Petrangeli 2017), in popular TV programmes (PiazzaPulita 2018), and in public protests (such as the ones they organised in Rome on 21 March 2017 and 24 February 2018). The topic of vaccines has also prominently featured the electoral campaign, which ended with the elections on 4 March 2018 and the electoral victory of the 5 Star Movement

(5SM) and the right-wing and anti-immigrant party Northern League—two political parties that later formed the coalition currently running the government. Both these parties—and particularly the 5SM—have challenged the new law on mandatory vaccines and have promised to repeal it once in power, thus returning to the 'old' system (Wheaton and Zampano 2018).[2]

Methodology

Data collection

Aggregated data was collected from Twitter utilising our custom Twitter Listener, built using the Python programming language. The Listener is designed to hook into Twitter's API and, based on a query, retrieve full tweet and related metadata from the past seven days, before monitoring Twitter's 'data hose' live for matching tweets. Our query sought to collect tweets containing any of the three tags, #novax, #libertadiscelta (transl.: 'freedom of choice') and #nonfiniscequi (transl: 'it doesn't end here'). These hashtags were the ones mostly used by the no-vax movement to express dissent against the Italian mandatory immunisation regime (especially the first one, #novax, see also Petrangeli 2017) and around which the no- and pro-vax debate has centred on Twitter. Collection took place in 2018, commencing on 2 February and ending 19 March, thus capturing the Twitter debate at the end of the electoral campaign and during and right after the Italian elections on 4 March 2018. During this time the Listener collected 9,735 tweets and retweets created between 23 January and the end date. The distribution of these tweets can be seen in the stacked area chart below (Figure 9.1), but across the entire dataset the collection was approximately 75% original tweets and 25% retweets.

The data collected was made available by users on a publicly accessible platform. The collection process retained only tweets that engaged with the #novax debate and network analysis treated users at an aggregate level. In outputs, researchers were careful to represent only the usernames of public figures who had a pre-existing public position prior to the debate analysed. The majority of users have not been identified, and instead their retweet and mention activity has been used in the production of the aggregated community mappings and measures. Given the focus of the collection on a single debate, it is also not possible to identify individual users purely by their interaction habits within this specific debate.

Identifying user communities

In order to identify whether there were any strong community of opinion within the users discussing #novax, a network was built based on both retweeting and mentioning behaviour, under the assumption that often (though not always) a retweet indicates endorsement and/or an indication that the content is considered important by the user, and mentioning indicates discourse between users (Ahn and Park 2015). Data from Twitter's API provides information both

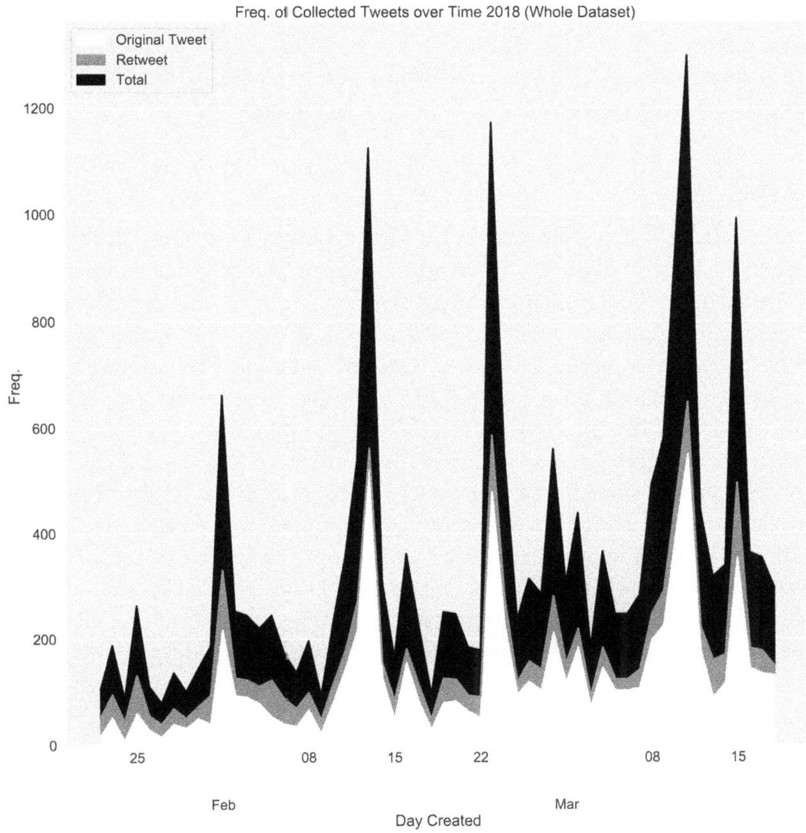

Figure 9.1 Frequency of tweets over time

on the source of a retweet as well as the presence of other user handles in text. This (aggregated) data was used to construct a directional network graph with individual users as the nodes, and a retweet or mention forming a directional edge. For retweets, the direction of the edge went from the original tweet user (edge source) to the user that retweeted them (edge target). This arrangement was chosen to better indicate influence and the spreading and reiteration of a common narrative. For interaction measures, the edge went from the user that initiated the interaction (edge source) to the user invoked in that tweet (edge target) for both retweets and mentions. This arrangement best represents the likelihood that an interaction is an act of engaging another user, and so the direction indicates the desire to engage with another user in the discourse. This graph data was then imported into Gephi for visualisation and further analysis. In particular we used Gephi's 'modularity' measure, an implementation of Blondel and colleagues' (2008) community detection algorithm, to determine whether particularly strong communities could be identified by retweeting behaviour. As noted by Ahn and Park (2015), retweeting is not just about the diffusion of information; it is also used to express agreement, form or maintain a social relationship, and share public anger. Retweeting is also more effective in diffusing information and forming communities around particular topics than forming longer-term reciprocal following relationships.

Data analysis

After establishing key communities and the network's overall structure, two measures of inter-community interaction were produced. These measures were used to identify the extent to which these key communities interacted across the group boundary between pro- and no-vax groups. The first measures the likelihood that a member of a group will be retweeted by someone outside of their group (e.g., a no-vaxxer's post by a pro-vax user and vice versa). The second measures the extent to which a member of each community is likely to mention a member of a different community. This was produced by first determining how many times the source of a connection (either the original retweet, or the writer of a tweet mentioning a user) was from a group different to that of the target (the original author of a retweeted tweet, or the user mentioned in the new tweet). This measure was then divided by the number of users within each community to provide an average likelihood of a user within group *x* either mentioning a user outside of group *x* or being retweeted by a user outside of group *x*.

In a second stage, involving a visual (Pink et al. 2016) and virtual ethnography of Twitter posts, we analysed the content (Altheide 1996) of the sampled tweets. Textual (e.g., newspaper articles, Facebook posts, blogs) and visual material (e.g., pictures, videos) referred to in the tweets has been included in the analysis up to one additional click. For concerns related to Twitter users' anonymity, we have decided not to use their personal identifiers (unless them being public figures), not to directly quote the content of the tweets (also see http://socialdatalab.net/ethics-resources), and not to reproduce the attached images. The findings of these analyses are reported below.

Findings

Network communities

Gephi's modularity measure indicated that within the network of 4,050 unique users that had either been involved in a retweeting or mentioning interaction (either as instigator or subject), there were 13 communities of more than five users. For visualisation, the network was distributed using Gephi's ForceAtlas 2 graph layout algorithm. Switching between retweet edges and mention edges before recalculating the position had little effect on the overall structure of the network, but did indicate closer relations between particular users in normally distant groups, a phenomenon addressed in greater detail below. Visual

Table 9.1 Frequency of unique users per group

Group	*Community*	*Freq. Unique Users*
Pro-vax	17	70
No-vax	0	67
Pro-vax	10	59
Pro-vax	36	37
Pro-vax	1	21
Pro-vax	71	13
No-vax	70	11

inspection of the graph indicated seven communities that were part of the two major components that had been established by the graph layout algorithm—No. 0, 1, 10, 17, 36, 70, and 71.

As shown in Figure 9.2, while communities No. 1, 10, 17, 36, and 71 form the group of pro-vaxxers, communities No. 0 and 70 constitute the group of no-vaxxers. Within these two groups, some individuals are more retweeted than others are. These individuals are graphically represented in Gephi (Figure 9.2) through nodes of medium and large size—the bigger the nodes, the more active the (re)tweeting habits of the relevant Twitter user(s). In the pro-vax communities (No. 1, 10, 17, 36, and 71) some of the most active individuals are Roberto Burioni, a scientist and university professor who has been very vocal on national media about the crucial role of vaccines for people's health and safety, the then Italian Minister of Health Beatrice Lorenzin, other private individuals, and medical doctors.

In the main no-vax community (No. 0), there are two main nodes whose tweets are substantially retweeted by the other users. While one of these two accounts uses a pseudonym, the second is the personal account of a journalist.

Figure 9.2 Network communities

Table 9.2 In- and outgroup interaction measures

Source side	*Kind*	*Ingroup interaction ratio*	*Outgroup interaction ratio*
No-vax	Mention	71.17	28.83
	Quote retweet	99.31	0.69
	Retweet	99.85	0.15
Pro-vax	Mention	84.55	15.45
	Quote retweet	99.57	0.43
	Retweet	99.97	0.03

Both users seem to be women and mothers. In community No. 70, we detected one main node, whose tweets published in English are retweeted by the main nodes of community No. 0.

Interaction—retweets and mentions

As illustrated in Table 9.2, the two groups of no- and pro-vaxxers show high degrees of ingroup interaction. This means that both no- and pro-vax people tend to retweet within their own ideological group: 99.85% and 99.97% of the retweets of no- and pro-vax people respectively are of people who think like them. The ratios for mentions are similar: 71% of the total mentions initiated by no-vaxxers and 84% of the mentions initiated by pro-vaxxers mention people belonging to their own ideological group. The interaction rates drop only when looking at the outgroup interaction ratio. Retweets between the two groups of no- and pro-vaxxers are on average extremely limited: only 0.15% of no-vaxxers' retweets are of pro-vaxxers' posts, and only 0.03% of pro-vaxxers retweets are of no-vax tweets. Mentions are also very limited, although seemingly higher from no-vax of pro-vax users: while 29% of no-vax mentions are of pro-vaxxers, the opposite only occurs in the 15.45% of the pro-vax mention cases. Although this data does not have statistical significance,[3] it seems to suggest that no-vax users are relatively more interactive than pro-vax users.

Content analysis

No-vax

Community No. 0: Twitter users belonging to this community—who refuse the label 'no-vax' for its negative connotations and mostly define themselves as 'concerned parents' and the 'people for the freedom of choice'—emphasise in their tweets the harms, and risks of harms, of children undergoing vaccination (particularly as regards the 10 vaccines made compulsory in Italy under the new law). Children are, in their views, treated like guinea pigs with the result of making them run the very high risk of getting cancer, leukaemia, and autoimmune diseases and increasing their likelihood of undergoing genetic mutations. Users provide 'evidence' of the risks and side effects of vaccines—which, in their opinion, are rather underplayed or denied by the government and the medical community—in many different ways. For instance, they make reference to journalistic investigations and parliamentary commissions on useless and cancer-related vaccines performed on the military and children (Iacovella 2012); conferences or film screenings discussing the side effects of vaccines, including through the voices of the affected 'victims' (RAVHPV 2016); media reports flagging the potential dangerousness of specific vaccines and the preoccupation of the medical association (RaiNews 2014); statements coming from (no-vax) doctors, including in books (Tarro 2018), online available public speeches (mostly of the no-vax activists Suzanne Humphries and Luc Montagnier), and open letters on the risks of vaccines (Montagnier and Joyeux 2018); scientific articles from which they wrongly deduced the link between vaccines and food allergies and autism; and stories of famous people refusing to vaccinate their children or being vocal about their negative attitudes towards mandatory vaccination schedules. Users also include references to the Italian law No. 210 of 25 February 1992, which envisages a compensation for individuals harmed by 'irreversible complications caused by compulsory vaccinations', and to cases in which courts have awarded damages for harms caused by vaccines on children.

In their tweets, users belonging to this community mostly speak about the new law, which introduces 10 mandatory vaccines for children. This law, in their opinion, is based on an 'invented' contingent epidemic of measles, and is mostly defined as 'dirty', 'criminal', 'murderous', and 'shameful'. It has been adopted against constitutional guarantees by a dictatorial and 'nazi' government and, by forbidding unvaccinated children to enrol to school, resonates the content of the racist laws in force in fascist Italy in 1938 against Jewish people. Also the removal of 'anti-vax' billboards of COMILVA (Coordination of the Italian Movement for the freedom of vaccinations) in some municipalities, which warned the public against the risks of vaccines (see Adinolfi (2018) and Triolo (2018)), has been described as in line with the fascist strategy of discriminating and hiding dissent. Many tweets are very critical towards the government, and particularly towards Minister of Health Beatrice Lorenzin. The only positive references to politicians are those related to the 5SM, which during the electoral campaign has been quite vocal about its opposition to the new law and, after the elections, is called on by users to keep its promises and repeal it.

The law is also seen as the result of the lobbying activities of Big Pharma, which aims at maximising the 'business' of vaccines. Science is not only seen as profit-driven but also as a 'religion': at least, some of its results are believed by the people with power without allowing any reasonable doubt. In line with the dominant literature on online misinformation on vaccines (e.g., Davies et al. 2002; Kata 2010, 2012; Betsch et al. 2012), a limited number of tweets published by the users of this community also explicitly talk about the existence of a conspiracy between the state and Big Pharma to create an 'unrealistic' need for more vaccines.

Worth highlighting is the fact that in most cases Twitter users belonging to this community firmly challenge the new law without, however, challenging the uselessness of vaccines. Mostly because of the risks involved, they ask to be free to decide—upon consultation with the family doctor and in the light of the case history and immune system of the child—whether to undergo vaccinations beyond those that were compulsory under the previous legislative framework (four, see endnote no. 1). These 'watered down' claims are typical in anti-vaxxers' online messages (Davies et al. 2002; Kata 2010, 2012; Betsch et al. 2012).

As reflected in their tweets, 'concerned parents' and relevant associations have organised many peaceful protests, including the one in Rome on 24 February 2018, and posted many tweets about them. Protests have been described as rather under-reported and 'censured' by the mainstream media (Pittelli 2018). According to the users of this community, protest has been silenced in many ways, including by taking off the billboards put on by COMILVA, with 'no-vax' organisers being prosecuted for 'false alarm' (Art. 658 penal code). Users also lament the circulation of leaflets inviting people to report the 'misinformation billboards' to the municipality, the police, the National Federation for the Orders of Medical Doctors and Dentists (FNOMCeO), and the relevant advertising agency. Also, a play called *The Decree* performed by the theatre company Investigative Artistic Theatre has been censured in many cities, including Bologna and Florence. Similarly, the screening of the movie *Vaxxed* by Andrew Wakefield (unveiling the disproven link between vaccines and autism) has been blocked in the city of Modena. For these users, repression has also been predicated on the isolation of the doctors who have been vocal or simply open about the risks and harms of vaccines, who in some cases have also lost their medical licence. This is in the face of the seemingly very widespread reluctance of doctors to administer vaccines to their patients because of their attached (high) risks and the doubts of the medical community (quotidianosanitá.it 2017).

Community No. 70: Most of the posts published by the users of community No. 70 are written in English and speak about the protest in Rome on 24 February, trying to gather support for it. Many of the Twitter posts of these users also talk about mandatory vaccines as the result of a conspiracy between Big Pharma and governments; the criminalisation and silencing of scientists who are critical of vaccines (e.g., of those who found vaccines contaminated by heavy metals); vaccines (particularly the hexavalent vaccine) as a 'torture'; and the freedom of choice.

Pro-vax

Community No. 1: The tweets posted by users in this community are very dismissive of the #novax movement. They regard them as 'bad people', 'shameless', 'ignorant', 'charlatans', 'liars', 'thugs', 'brainless', and so forth. No-vaxxers are mainly considered a-scientific: they are described as a group of incompetent people (mostly moms) who pretend to be and act as doctors. In particular, no-vaxxers are accused of wrongly reading and interpreting scientific studies; denying established scientific results (e.g., that autism is not caused by vaccines, and that vaccines are actually helpful to avoid and prevent epidemics); and using homeopathy and other untested practices (e.g., vitamin C to 'cure' cancer) instead of recognised medical treatments. As a result, these users call for the termination of no-vaxxers' parental rights and for the exclusion of no-vax politicians (5SM) from politics.

Community No. 10: Similar to the users belonging to community No. 1, also in this case users—and, particularly, both laypeople and public figures like Roberto Burioni and the war surgeon and NGO Emergency founder Gino Strada—tend to insult no-vax people. They are considered 'stupid', 'idiots', 'brainless', 'ignorant', 'criminals', 'murderers', 'selfish' and 'dangerous', as they take decisions of not vaccinating their children that are potentially harmful for the other vaccinated children and for unvaccinated kids with autoimmune diseases. In support of this, they include figures and other evidence (mostly derived from newspaper articles, e.g., Salvatori 2018) suggesting a substantial increase of measles in 2017 and the re-emergence of old and eradicated diseases. No-vax doctors believing in homeopathic treatments are also considered 'charlatans', 'shameless speculators', and 'dangerous'. No-vax positions are also associated with the Northern League and with the 5SM, which are both seen as regressive ('anti-science', 'populist', 'anti-euro', anti-Europe) and authoritarian ('fascist') political parties. Members of this community, in particular through the voice of Roberto Burioni, tend to antagonise the 5SM (DiRE 2018); they also tend to be supporters of the then government run by the Democratic Party (with Gentiloni premier), calling for the firm application ('zero tolerance') of the ministerial decree on vaccines.

Community No. 17: In addition to calling no-vax people 'dumb' and 'ignorant' and talking about their protest on 24 February in very dismissive terms, users of this community mostly speak about the instrumental use of the #novax campaign by the 5SM and the Northern League during the electoral campaign to get consensus among the no-vax people at the expense of children's health. They call these tactics 'the worse possible', 'the most unethical', 'slimy', and 'disgusting'. Similar to the users of community No. 17, these users also seem to be supportive of Democratic Party and of the mandatory immunisation regime introduced under the Gentiloni government.

Community No. 36: The particularity of this community is that users in their tweets talk much about the 'no-vax' billboards in many Italian cities, which show children allegedly dead because of vaccines (for an example, see Bellizzi 2018). They second the initiative of the medical board of the city of Foggia to report the billboards to the authorities, and describe the billboards with dead children as 'sordid' and a 'horror', and no-vax people as 'jackals'.

Community No. 71: Users belonging to this community mostly write in German addressing a case of allegedly fake news involving Reinhold Holzer, a no-vax activist of the Alto Adige/Süd Tirol Province, who suggested the existence of a correlation between the injection of vaccines to a 4-year-old and his emergency hospitalisation a few days later. Twitter posts also mention the case of Bolzano (the chief town of the previously mentioned province, also called a 'no-vax stronghold') where many children are un-immunised and where politicians tend to discourage parents from immunising their children (Ansa.it 2018).

Discussion and conclusive thoughts

In line with the research on conversations and debates on Twitter, which emphasises their polarised nature (Gunnarsson Lorentzen 2014), the social network analysis performed in this study revealed little to no interaction between the two groups of pro- and anti-vaxxers on Twitter. Users tend to retweet (and thus endorse) tweets posted by users belonging to their own 'ideological' group. This notwithstanding, no-vaxxers seem to be more prone than pro-vaxxers to mention people outside their group. Little engagement with each other's arguments has also been found through the content analysis of the sampled tweets and their attached textual and visual material.

No-vax messages are very diverse in their content. In line with the dominant literature on online misinformation on vaccines (e.g., Davies et al. 2002; Kata 2010, 2012; Betsch et al. 2012), they cover conspiratorial claims framing vaccines as the results of the entangled interests of Big Pharma and governments; an emphasis on the harms of vaccines mostly proven by more or less 'scientific' evidence (including privately published material, alternative medicine press, and misinterpreted journal articles) and anecdotal accounts; and 'watered down' messages that are not oppositional towards vaccines but in favour of the 'freedom of choice'. Contrary to the public health literature on anti-vaxxers' messages on the Web and Facebook (Smith and Graham 2017), emotive stories only rarely feature the content of Twitter posts (for an example of victims speaking at a conference, see RAVHPV 2016). In addition, the 'people for the freedom of choice' also lament the suppression of their parental rights and right to informed consent, the criminalisation of their dissent (Rawlinson 2017), and their silencing by an authoritarian regime through removed billboards, cancelled events, media underreporting, and criminal charges filed against activists.

The messages of pro-vaxxers—including by public figures within them, such as the scientist and university professor Roberto Burioni—tend to be more homogeneous, dismissive, and disparaging in their content: opponents are reduced to regressive individuals who distrust science and refuse to immunise their children, preferring to inject them with harmful substances or homeopathic treatments at most, which have the only effect of causing their death and harm to others (who are vaccinated or cannot be vaccinated because of their serious medical history). Very much neglected are, however, the *rights-based* arguments used by no-vaxxers to motivate their resistance and doubts towards a tough mandatory immunisation regime for children (with six newly introduced mandatory vaccines and tough sanctions in case of non-compliance), which is seen as excessively constraining parental rights and the right to informed consent, much emphasised in public health treatments in recent years. It is worth highlighting here the fact that the effectiveness of a rather 'aggressive' and unidirectional method of communication by science advocates (Burioni, in this case) has been highly debated in recent years, and that the literature on science and technology communication mostly emphasises the importance of establishing a dialogue between scientists and the public, with the latter being also engaged with science and science communication (Bucchi and Trench 2014).

Italy is a country with high medical illiteracy (Duffy 2018) and high levels of hesitancy towards vaccines (Napolitano et al. 2018), which has also been proven by the recent general elections and the electoral victory of the two populist political parties (5SM and Northern League) that opposed the mandatory immunisation regime introduced in 2017. In this context, issuing dismissive online messages may not be the best strategy to counter vaccine-related misinformation and raise national vaccine coverage, and may exacerbate and maintain pre-existing polarisations. In line with previous studies (Love et al. 2013; Tafuri et al. 2014), enhancing communication and interaction also on social media by better trained public figures may be the way forward, along with increasing public confidence in the health system (Gualano et al. 2018).

Notes

1 The four mandatory vaccines before the legislative change were to protect against polio, diphtheria, tetanus, and hepatitis B.

2 Only recently, however, the founder of the 5SM, Beppe Grillo, has signed a pact in defence of science, and against pseudoscience, drafted by Roberto Burioni. This has generated much criticism from the 5SM's members who are against immunisation practices for children. Grillo replied to this criticism by saying that he is critical towards the mandatory nature of vaccines, which is a political matter; not against vaccines themselves, which when safe and effective are the product of science (*LaRepubblica* 2019).

3 Whilst the differences between no-vax and pro-vax in the proportion of outgroup interaction for retweets was shown to be significant (p: 0.004) this is to be expected due to the use of retweets to form the initial communities. The differences between groups for outgroup mentioning behaviour was not statistically significant (p: 0.062) but close, and could be attributed to the low sample of interacting users.

References

Adinolfi C (2018) Vaccini, manifesti no-vax ad Arezzo e Viareggio. *La Repubblica*. Mar 10. Available at: http://firenze.repubblica.it/cronaca/2018/03/10/news/vaccini_manifesti_no-vax_ad_arezzo_e_viareggio-190922372/

Ahn H and Park JH (2015) The structural effects of sharing function on Twitter networks: focusing on the retweet function. *Journal of Information Science* 41(3):354–365

Altheide D (1996) *Qualitative media analysis*. Thousand Oaks, CA: Sage

Ansa.it (2018) Lorenzin, bimbi senza vaccini non finiranno l'anno scolastico. *Ansa*. Feb 28. Available at: www.ansa.it/canale_saluteebenessere/notizie/medicina/2018/02/28/lorenzin-sanzioni-a-chi-non-vaccina-per-ideologia_59f04b0b-774a-4584–8ab6-bd5f1de7d23a.html

Bellizzi T (2018) 'Sono un bambino morto dopo il vaccino'. E i medici di Foggia si indignano per il manifesto no vax. *La Repubblica.* Jan 23. Available at: https://bari.repubblica.it/cronaca/2018/01/23/news/_sono_un_neonato_morto_dopo_il_vaccino_a_foggia_l_ordine_dei_medici_denuncia_il_manifesto_no_vax-187116944/

Betsch C, Brewer NT, Brocard P, Davies P, Gaissmaier W, Haase N, Leask J, Renkewitz F, Renner B, Reyna VF, Rossmann C, Sachse K, Schachinger A, Siegrist M and Stryk M (2012) Opportunities and challenges of Web 2.0 for vaccination decisions, *Vaccine* 30(25):3727–3733

Blondel V, Guillaume J, Lambiotte R and Lefebvre E (2008) Fast unfolding of communities in large networks. *Journal of Statistical Mechanics: Theory and Experiment* 10:1–12

Blume S (2006) Anti-vaccination movements and their interpretations. *Social Science & Medicine* 62(3):628–642

Bucchi M and Trench B (2014) Science and communication research: themes and challenges. In Bucchi M and Trench B (eds.) *Routledge handbook of public communication of science and technology.* London: Routledge

Constitutional Court (2018) Judgment No 5 of 18 January 2018. Available at: www.cortecostituzionale.it/actionSchedaPronuncia.do?anno=2018&numero=4

Davies P, Chapman S and Leask J (2002) Antivaccination activists on the world wide web. *Archives of Disease in Childhood* 87(1):22–25

DiRE (2018) Vaccini, Burioni: 'Per capolista M5S sono un genocidio. Stia lontana dalla politica'. Feb 1. Available at: www.dire.it/01-02-2018/169595-vaccini-burioni-per-capolista-m5s-sono-un-genocidio-stia-lontana-dalla-politica/

Duffy B (2018) Autism and vaccines: more than half of people in Britain, France, Italy still think there may be a link. *The Conversation.* Aug 22. Available at: https://theconversation.com/autism-and-vaccines-more-than-half-of-people-in-britain-france-italy-still-think-there-may-be-a-link-101930

Gualano MR, Bert F, Voglino G, Buttinelli E, D'Errico MM, De Waure C, Di Giovanni P, Fantini MP, Giuliani AR, Marranzano M and Masanotti G (2018) Attitudes towards compulsory vaccination in Italy: results from the NAVIDAD multicentre study. *Vaccine* 36(23):3368–3374

Gunnarsson Lorentzen D (2014) Polarisation in political Twitter conversations. *Aslib Journal of Information Management* 66(3):329–341

Iacovella V (2012) Vaccinazioni sbagliate e fatte male dietro i tumori dei soldati italiani. *La Repubblica.* Oct 6. Available at: http://inchieste.repubblica.it/it/repubblica/rep-it/2012/10/06/news/vaccini-44012069/

ISS (2017) *Morbillo in Italia: bollettino settimanale.* Available at: www.epicentro.iss.it/problemi/morbillo/Infografica2017.asp

Kata A (2010) A postmodern Pandora's box: anti-vaccination misinformation on the internet. *Vaccine* 28(7):1709–1716

Kata A (2012) Anti-vaccine activists, Web 2.0, and the postmodern paradigm: an overview of tactics and tropes used online by the anti-vaccination movement. *Vaccine* 30(25): 3778–3789

La Repubblica (2019) Grillo firma il patto pro-vax di Burioni: "Io contro? Polemica da terrapiattisti". E Di Maio prende le distanze. Available at: www.repubblica.it/politica/2019/01/10/news/grillo_firma_con_renzi_il_patto_pro-vax_di_burioni-216233394/

Lavorgna A and Di Ronco A (2017) Fraud victims or unwary accomplices? An exploratory study of online communities supporting quack medicine. In Van Duyne PC, Harvey J, Antonopoulos GA and Von Lampe K (eds.) *The many faces of crime for profit and ways of tackling it.* Nijmegen, NL: Wolf Legal Publishers

Love B, Himelboim I, Holton A and Stewart K (2013) Twitter as a source of vaccination information: content drivers and what they are saying. *American Journal of Infection Control* 41(6):568–570

Montagnier L and Joyeux H (2018) Appello alla Ragione. 11 vaccini: Appello urgente al personale e ai professionisti della sanità. Available at: http://telegra.ph/APPELLO-ALLA-RAGIONE-01-24

Napolitano F, D'Alessandro A and Angelillo IF (2018) Investigating Italian parents' vaccine hesitancy: a cross-sectional survey. *Human Vaccines & Immunotherapeutics* 14(7):1–8

Olpiński M (2012) Anti-vaccination movement and parental refusals of immunization of children in USA. *Pediatria Polska* 87(4):381–385

Petrangeli G (2017) #NoVax, la rete si organizza contro i vaccini. *Huffington Post*. Aug 10. Available at: www.huffingtonpost.it/guido-petrangeli/novax-la-rete-si-organizza-contro-i-vaccini_a_23057407/

PiazzaPulita (2018) Non Gioco più. Episode of Mar 15. Available at: www.youtube.com/watch?v=uGuAoM0lgv0

Pink S, Horst H, Postill J, Hjorth L, Lewis T and Tacchi J (2016) *Digital ethnography: principles and practice*. London: Sage

Pittelli T (2018) Libera scelta vaccinale, la marea di genitori a Roma ignorata dai tg. Ecco le loro storie. *L'esuberante – mamma reporter*. Feb 28. Available at: www.lesuberante.it/libera-scelta-vaccinale-la-marea-genitori-roma-ignorata-dai-tg-le-storie/

quotidianosanitá.it (2017) Vaccini. Un sanitario su tre non ci crede e teme gli effetti collaterali. I risultati di una survey on line presentati oggi a Pisa. Mar 27. Available at: www.quotidianosanita.it/lavoro-e-professioni/articolo.php?articolo_id=49202

RaiNews (2014) Caso vaccini, morti sospette. Due casi a Roma. Aperte inchieste in Toscana. Available at: www.rainews.it/dl/rainews/articoli/Caso-vaccini-aumentano-le-segnalazioni-sospette-ad672fcb-2d8b-415e-9f19-f7fcc2b43a58.html

RAVHPV (2016) Vaccino HPV – La testimonianza delle ragazze danneggiate. Available at: www.youtube.com/watch?v=Rs6u7QdCm3M&feature=youtu.be

Rawlinson P (2017) Immunity and impunity: corruption in the state-pharma nexus. *International Journal for Crime, Justice and Social Democracy* 6(4):86–99

Sak G, Diviani N, Allam A and Schulz PJ (2016) Comparing the quality of pro-and anti-vaccination online information: a content analysis of vaccination-related webpages. *BMC Public Health* 16(1):38

Salvatori C (2018) Il morbillo torna a far paura Lazio record, 1.699 casi. *Il Corriere della Sera*. Jan 29. Available at: https://roma.corriere.it/digital-edition/CORRIEREFC_ROMANA_WEB/2018/01/29/6/il-morbillo-torna-a-far-paura-lazio-record-1699-casi_U43430379619522vYH.shtml

Smith N and Graham T (2017) Mapping the anti-vaccination movement on Facebook. *Information, Communication & Society* 21:1–18

Tafuri S, Gallone MS, Cappelli MG, Martinelli D, Prato R and Germinario C (2014) Addressing the anti-vaccination movement and the role of HCWs. *Vaccine* 32(38):4860–4865

Tarro G (2018) *Dieci cose da sapere sui vaccini: Tutta la verita': Un libero indispensabile per genitori consapevoli*. Rome: Newton Compton

Triolo G (2018) Manifesti 'no vax' in città: 'Pizzarotti li faccia rimuovere. *ParmaReport*. Jan 15. Available at: www.parmareport.it/manifesti-no-vax-citta-pizzarotti-li-faccia-rimuovere/

Vernon JG (2003) Immunisation policy: from compliance to concordance? *British Journal of General Practice* 53(490):399–404

Vicari S (2013) Public reasoning around social contention: a case study of Twitter use in the Italian mobilization for global change. *Current Sociology* 61:474–490

Ward A (2016) Vaccines are among Big Pharma's best-selling products: expansion of immunisation programmes in developing countries lifts market. *Financial Times*. Apr 25. Available at: www.ft.com/content/93374f4a-e538-11e5-a09b-1f8b0d268c39

Wheaton S and Zampano G (2018) Vaccines debate gives Italian elections a shot in the arm. *Politico*. Feb 14. Available at: www.politico.eu/article/vaccine-debate-gives-italian-election-campaign-a-shot-in-the-arm/

World Health Organisation (2019) Ten threats to global health in 2019. Available at: www.who.int/emergencies/ten-threats-to-global-health-in-2019

10 Traditional herbal medicine and the challenges of pharmacovigilance

Nayeli Urquiza-Haas and Emilie Cloatre

Introduction

Herbal medicines, especially those sold through online pharmacies, have been the focus of criticism, particularly by those who argue the herbal medicinal market is not regulated strictly enough to protect the public from 'fake' and dangerous products (McIntyre 2011). However, the regulation of herbal medicines in general raises significant challenges. By their nature, herbal medicines tend to sit at the border of the regulation of medicine and at the border of public imaginaries of what 'real' medicines are. Governments have gradually recognised the significance of herbal medicines in traditional healing systems and how they represent key sources of primary health care across regions (WHO 2013). Yet herbal medicines are difficult to regulate, both because of the way in which herbs can circulate and because of their inscription in multiple epistemological systems. While details about regulatory approaches vary, a common position taken by regulators and policy makers, notably in the EU, is that herbal medicines are potentially effective, yet should abide by comparable (if adjusted) standards of safety, quality, and efficacy applied to all medicinal products (WHO 2000; Li 2002; Walker 2015). Without those standards, critics argue that herbal remedies run the risk of being harmless placebos or potentially dangerous products (Ernst 1998; Derbyshire 2000). At the same time, herbal medicines belong to circuits of care that differ from those of other medicines. In part, this is because of cultural bounds and because their practitioners predominantly do not belong to the biomedical communities. But it is also because the suspicion they attract means that regulators do not always see them as 'real' medicines (and therefore ill-suited to the systems of funding or distribution that those may rely upon).

Arguably, herbal products straddle the real/fake boundary of pharmaceuticals: they are, at best, at the edge of the medicinal circuit. But while herbal medicines as a whole are never fully 'true' medicines in the eyes of the regulatory system, 'fake' herbal medicines remain a key concern for regulators. Indeed, discussions about facilitating the circulation of herbal medicines are often held back by the fear that opening up their market would facilitate the entry of fake or dangerous products (Sénat 2018: 70). Such 'fake' herbal medicines can cover a range of situations such as the use of mislabelled, poorly identified plants or plant-parts, adulterated products, or contaminated products. Concern may extend by association to unauthorised products that are neither dangerous nor 'fake', which, as we will see, raises other dilemmas. It is true that people have died or have had their health severely compromised by adulterated herbal remedies. This has resulted in bans against the sale and importation of some plants used in traditional medicine systems and in non-traditional formulations sold in the wellness market (Corns and Metcalfe 2002). At the same time, the distrust towards plants risks displacing them to the margins, where they persist yet as illegal substances in illicit or unregulated market spaces. Thus, regulatory regimes for herbal medicines require a careful balance that has proven difficult to strike: while regulating herbal medicines is necessary and ensuring that those that are sold are of a certain quality and are what they claim to be, restricting the range of what is available onto the market too much may not be desirable if patients are driven to unregulated spaces instead (Corazza et al. 2014). In addition, mechanisms currently in place to regulate which herbal products can enter regulated markets have been criticised for facilitating the systems of some herb medicines (notably, those with established local use) over others (in particular those traditional medicines or herbal substances imported from China) (Virtosu 2018).

Of course, the weeding out of fake or dangerous medicines, including herbal product, cannot be done exclusively at the point of market authorisation: much of it happens through pharmacovigilance mechanisms, once products are put onto the market. Here, however, the ambivalent position of herbal medicines is problematic. Safety mechanisms have been predominantly directed at 'real' medicines, not 'fake' ones, resulting in a failure to fully engage with herbals, beyond those that have entered the western biomedical paradigm by extracting their active components (e.g., acetylsalicylic acid from willow bark). Part of the reason, as we will argue, is that herbal products belong to socio-technical assemblages of care (Puig and Bellacasa 2011) that are not fully acknowledged or considered by regulators, both in the regulation of products and in pharmacovigilance mechanisms. In the end, herbal medicines are a useful site from which to explore how different modalities of care and their relative power (Martin et al. 2015) continue to influence the regulation of therapeutics, including in Europe, which is the focus of this chapter.

We suggest 'fakeness' functions as a discursive tool that polices the boundaries between 'real' medicines and non-conventional medicines, yet as one that is fundamentally ill-adapted to acknowledging the complexity of regulating herbal medicines and the limits of existing regulations. To that extent, we point out the difficulties encountered by a law that aims to disentangle 'real' from 'fake' medicines when ordering alternative therapeutic materials that do not rely (or do not rely exclusively) on scientific knowledge. Drawing on Science and Technology Studies (STS), we query the assumptions underpinning notions of safety and evidence in the law regarding herbal and traditional medicines. We ultimately suggest that regulations continue to be entangled in persisting epistemological imbalances premised around a science versus culture binary, which ultimately limits the possibility for various actors to contribute to shared definitions of what constitutes legitimate or illegitimate alternatives in medicine. We draw on literature in the field, government reports, as well as preliminary data from 15 semi-structured interviews with regulators, herbalists, and herbalists' associations conducted over the course of our research on the regulation of traditional medicine in the United Kingdom and France.

Are herbal medicines 'real medicines' for the law?

Herbal and traditional medicines are used widely across the world and represent an important first line of care in low- to middle-income countries. Around 80% of people in developing countries rely on traditional medicines (WHO 2002), which often include plant-based medicines. In Europe, patients also turn to 'natural' products for a variety of reasons, sometimes considering them safer than allopathic medicines. In the EU alone, the herbal medicinal product market surpasses that of prescription medicines (Ruiz-Poveda 2015), and research suggests the demand for 'natural' products in industrialised countries has been growing steadily (Pickup and Hodges 2002). Products originate from a range of cultural and epistemological healing systems, from local folk medicine to more established traditional medical systems (Ayurveda, Chinese, Unani, Tibetan). They also make a wide range of health claims: from weight loss to erectile dysfunction, female hormonal issues, colds, depression, sleep disorders, digestive issues, or in some cases cancer (in relation both to the alleviation of side effects from treatment and, more controversially, to curative claims).

Herbal products also come in all sorts of forms and are not necessarily commercialised products. Some may be collected in the wild, prepared at home in the form of teas, or even consumed as food-stuff for medicinal purposes. What constitutes a 'medicine' per se varies depending on the medical knowledge system one is alluding to: most traditions do not separate food-stuff from medicines (Cocks and Valerie 2002; Langwick 2018). In contrast, western modern medicine and its regulation have relied on stricter categories that define what is or is not a medicine through the framework of biomedicine and pharmacology that emerged in the late 19th and the 20th centuries (Jackson 2012). This is shaped largely by the so-called magic bullet or wonder drug model of drug discovery geared around finding one active compound capable of hitting a single physiological target (and, often, capable of being patented) (e.g., curing a disease) (Porter 1999; Gaudillière 2002).

A notable feature of herbal medicines in law is that a majority of them are not 'quite medicine': they are entangled in both special regulatory regimes and their own circuits of distribution (though how those are organised varies from country to country within the EU). In addition, plant-based medicines are frequently under attack in public discourses for not being 'real' medicines, meaning they are commonly associated to being 'placebo' products (Wahlberg 2008). For example, a 2017 consultation by NHS England characterised herbal medicine and homeopathy as 'low-medical value' products to be included in a prescription black-list (NHS England 2017). As another example, a UK government report singled out traditional Chinese and Ayurvedic medicines as a group of non-conventional healing that 'favour a philosophical approach and are indifferent to the scientific principles of conventional medicine' (House of Lords 2000, para. 2.1). For herbal medicines to be fully considered as 'medicines', they need to obtain biomedical legitimation, including through multi-phase clinical trials. The many products that do not, either because their efficacy is insufficiently proven or because they cannot be isolated from the healing system that surrounds them for the purpose of clinical testing (Evans 2008), are relocated to the boundary of health and wellbeing, medicines, and food.

Legally, in the EU, the most common pathways onto the market are either as Traditional Herbal Medicinal Products (THMP) under Directive 2004/24/EC or under EU Food Law (Regulation (EC) No. 178/2002) and Directive 2002/46/EC on Food Supplements. In this chapter, we focus primarily on the former. Such regulation has focused on protecting the public by enforcing quality and safety standards, and to some extent, proof of efficacy (Pickup and Hodges 2002; Ruiz-Poveda 2015). Through these regimes, EU regulation offers at least some herbal medicines (those that can be proven to have been used 'traditionally' for at least 15 years in the EU or 30 years outside the EU) a particular regime, much lighter than the marketing authorisation procedures used for other medicines. Chinese and Ayurvedic stakeholders, however, have observed that the regime is less adapted to their own traditions and practices. First, the time requirement places some barriers specifically for their (imported) practices, as applications need to prove long-time use *within* the EU (Fan et al. 2012). Second, the reliance of the system on a choice between a regime of food and a regime of traditional medicines does not correspond to all healing systems (and is arguably very western in its assumptions) (Porter 1999; Saks 2002; Ijaz et al. 2016). Third, the regime makes it more difficult for mixtures that contain multiple plants, or indeed a mixture of plants and animal or mineral products, to be approved. From the outset, the system therefore appears less inclusive of non-western epistemological approaches to healing.

Applications for THMP status rely on approval or previous inclusion of a plant in the European Union Herbal Monographs and List Entries administered by the European Medicines Agency (EMA) or the pharmacopeias of the member state. Inclusion in the EMA monographs is decided by the Committee of Herbal Medicines Products, empowered to assess scientifically the safety and efficacy of herbal substances, preparations, and combinations. A fundamental aspect of the monographs is that the safety and quality of products is upheld through correct identification of the plant to avoid contamination from another species or a completely different genus. Identification relies more these days on technology (light microscopy and DNA barcoding) than on observation of the morphological and chemical features of a plant (Barnes 2003), a development which also could potentially affect the practice of herbalists who often grow or rely on other ways to identify the plant (sight, taste, etc.).

Bearing in mind these issues, what is most significant about the THMP directive is that it recognises that the effectiveness of a medicine may be assessed on the basis of 'traditional' use and therefore gives plant-based medicines that have not undergone the costly and extensive multi-phase clinical trials a regulated access to the market, although through a particular 'not quite medicines' regime. However, herbalists argue that the regime is still restrictive and not in line with the way herbal products are 'traditionally' used (Whitehouse 2014). For example, polyherbal combinations do not fit easily within the parameters relied on by the EU medicines regulation (including THMP) to assess proof of quality and safety (Quah 2003; Evans 2008). Ayurvedic and traditional Chinese medicine formulations that include non-herbal ingredients (for example, substances of animal origin, such as ghee) or herbs cannot be approved under the current regime (something that has been accommodated for pharmaceuticals, but not for 'Traditional Herbal Remedies'). In the end, some associations have complained that the directive limits ingredients to only plant-based substances, and manufacturers have had to alter polyherbal formulations, including reducing the number of herbs used, in order to comply with the registration requirements (Alliance for Natural Health International 2013). Overall, to enter the EU market, even traditional herbal medicines that successfully get approved under the THMP regime have to undergo a process of translation and inscription through the legal-scientific technologies (laboratory tests and regulations) to fit the medico-legal regulatory system and be considered as sufficiently safe, proven, and 'real' (as a THMP if not as a medicine) (Kim 2007). However, at the end of the process, THMPs are never 'fully' proven according to the standards required for allopathic medicines, and to that extent the THMP regime implies these herbal medicines are only 'potentially' effective since they are based on traditional knowledge rather than 'science'. According to the directive, THMPs are considered 'not harmful under the specific conditions of use and the pharmacological effects and efficacy are plausible based on long-term use and of available experience'.[1] This is characteristic of the ambivalence that is core to the place of herbal medicines in healthcare more generally and feeds into the difficulty of weeding out 'fake' herbal remedies. While tradition offers them a legal route to prove their (a priori) safety, this is not sufficient to prove their efficacy as medicines and therefore inscribe them into the health system under the same conditions (Barnes 2003; Scarborough and Fernandes 2011). As a result, they are safe enough to be sold in most cases without prescription (as we return to, without necessarily remaining grounded in the traditional practices that demonstrated their safety), but not proven enough to occupy a defined place within the health system itself.

In practice, conditions of sale and distribution vary from country to country. In the UK, herbal products tend to be sold in health shops and pharmacies over the counter, without prescription-only medicines (POM) controls. Moreover, without full proof of effectiveness, THMPs are relegated to the space of chronic disease and minor illnesses, like colds, where allopathic medicine might not be so successful or where interventions cost more (i.e., antibiotics). That being said, there are some exceptions in the conditions of sale for more hazardous plants, available as POMs which only registered herbalists or pharmacists can deliver by following conditions set out in the law (i.e., limited quantities or mode of use) (Melvin 2013). In France, the situation is different as THMPs fall under the monopoly of pharmacists, and therefore can only be sold by them. However, the training of both pharmacists and doctors does not include extensive engagement with herbal medicines, limiting chances of traditional knowledge becoming part of the distribution system. Herbalists, who often practice on the border of il/legality, insist that this means that the advice patients will be given is often more limited than what 'expert herbalists' would provide. Indeed, unofficial opportunities to access such advice and products outside of the pharmacy sector abound, online as well as offline. In practice, in both contexts, traditional herbal medicines sit awkwardly as both medicinal products of a kind and 'not quite' medicines, in circuits that are neither quite biomedical nor quite those of traditional healing.

Finally, despite attempts to regulate traditional (herbal) products more strictly and their progressive integration into the European market as THMP (European Medicines Agency 2017), others continue to the enter as food supplements, sold in both licit and illicit online pharmacies or by herbal medicine practitioners (Corns and Metcalfe 2002; Silano et al. 2011; Biagi et al. 2016). Regulatory hurdles are lighter for food supplements than for medicines, and the main compromise is the inability to make therapeutic claims on their products. However, because some 'health claims' can be made on food supplements, this compromise is relatively modest and the thin distinction between health and therapeutic claims entrenches yet further the liminality of herbal products. This liminality affects how 'fake' herbal products can be dealt with by the law, including how pharmacovigilance systems identify fake herbal medicines. We turn to these issues in the next section.

Faking in plant-medicine: regulation and displacement

Aristolochia is a large plant genus with about 500 species spread across the world. Its medicinal use dates back to 5th-century China, but it was also common in the Greek, Roman, and Byzantine pharmacopeia where, according to Scarborough and Fernandes (2011), ancient writers often misidentified the effects of these plants. In the 1990s, importation and use of these plants was banned in Europe after reported cases of liver and kidney damage in Belgium and the UK (Peralta et al. 2016). *Aristolochia* has stood as a cautionary tale about how traditional knowledge systems are badly placed in issues of public health safety. Yet, a potential problem of general medicines regime is that it monitors less stringently these types of products in comparison to licensed medicines, particularly POMs. Rather than a problem of market authorisation, this is one of pharmacovigilance, which plants, as 'not quite medicine', can more easily escape. Domestic and regional regulators as well as international bodies (WHO) rely in great part on pharmacovigilance systems to identify potential sources of risk.

Pharmacovigilance systems mine data of adverse reactions and analyse potential risks through science (European Commission 2019).

In the context of THMP, the 2004 directive also creates a legal obligation on manufacturers to report adverse effects of herbal medicine. However, the weeding out of 'fake herbal medicines' may not be given quite the attention it deserves because, as those products fall outside the main health system, they also fall outside clear regimes of reporting. To some extent, pharmacovigilance is ill-equipped to handle the particularity of herbal medicines and their co-existence with conventional medicine. This means that while the test of time is factored in safety assessments in the pre-marketing phase, adverse effects from herb-herb or herb-drug interactions arise only once these medications are out in the market. Adverse effects may also arise from unlicensed formulations sold online that surface only when they are serious enough that they force people to seek medical assistance. However, patients tend to assume that herbal medicines are in general safe and/or, when they self-medicate in plants, do not disclose the use of herbal medicines because of fear that the GP will recommend discontinuing use (Green et al. 2006).

Beyond the context of self-medication, herbalists may not always be in a position to feed into the public health care system. In the UK, the law allows their practices to exist, yet without any formal links to the NHS, complicating modes of communication (Maclennan and Pendry 2011). In France, because herbalists often operate illegally (as the distribution of herbal medicines is predominantly under the monopoly of pharmacists), they are not always in a position to, or willing to, engage with doctors. Finally, the restrictions placed on the range or type of products that can be given THMP status means that some herbalists will sell or import products that, in principle, are prohibited. For example, practitioners of Ayurvedic and Chinese traditions in the UK bring herbs in their personal suitcase or get them from online suppliers. From the view of directors of professional herbalist associations, therein lies the risk of encountering bad batches, contaminated with toxic bio-organisms or substances (Interviews 12.11.2018 and 30.05.2018). Illegality makes both the circulation of product less visible and therefore less safe and their reporting less likely. In effect, scepticism towards herbal medicines and the intrinsic biomedical approach in regulation facilitates a space for parallel healing practices, disconnected from biomedical health care systems, where herbalists may operate on the edge of the law or fully illegally. When they do so, they see themselves as having to cope with a system that makes it impossible for patients to obtain bona fide products, and may describe their own illegal activities as 'safer' than the obvious alternative of online purchases. To manage these issues collectively, some associations such as the National Institute of Medical Herbalists (Huntley et al. 2005; HMAC 2014) have and are developing internal pharmacovigilance and quality assurance mechanisms (e.g., building a list of approved suppliers), while the British Herbal Medicines Association and the Register of Chinese Herbal Medicines recommend members to follow a list of approved suppliers (BHMA 2019; RCHM 2019). These efforts, however, remain hindered by the marginality of the practice itself (Barnes 2003). In the following section, we illustrate how the challenge of weeding out herbal medicines has been complicated by the effacement of medicinal plants' epistemological and social practices of care, which are themselves embedded to the traditional medicine knowledges from which they emerged.

Knowledges and pharmacovigilance: uprooting 'toxic' herbs

Regulators find themselves in a conundrum: legitimising herbal medicines is made difficult by a fear of 'fakes' infiltrating the market, yet finding a solution is complicated by their location at the edge of the health system. Fakes are at the core of calls for tighter regulation, yet uncertainty around fakes also participates in the wariness against facilitating the broader distribution of herbal medicines as a whole and their fuller embracing in healthcare. We argue that they also signal a significant point of crisis in regulatory knowledge: both the regulation of licensed herbal medicines and the pharmacovigilance regimes that surround them are affected by such knowledge issues: without fully engaging the types of knowledge that herbal medicines rely upon and recognising the space they occupy in health practices, designing a well-functioning vigilance system is less feasible. Nonetheless, regulatory regimes so far have decoupled herbs from the cultural webs in which they are entangled to such an extent that traditional practitioners are rarely trusted as potential actors of the vigilance system.

While the practical considerations for such debates are significant, ideological tensions should not be under-estimated. Developing legitimate circuits for the distribution of herbal medicines always hits itself against the broader question of whether they belong at all to the healthcare system. Notwithstanding the presence of criminal fraudulent practices, caution is warranted when it comes to how discourse on the safety of health products mobilise legal categories against the supply of banned substances, as the latter tend to be punctuated by racism and gendered notions of criminality (Seddon 2016; Urquiza-Haas 2017). For example, Laura Foster shows how advertisement of *hoodia* (a stem succulent), traditionally used by the San people in South Africa and marketed in the global herbal diet industry, reifies histories of colonialism and embeds them in contemporary neoliberal projects that position knowledge-ownership as a driver of economic innovation. Drawing on feminist techno-science studies, she argues that the commercial pharmaceutical model, which relies on defining ownership through patents, is underpinned by a gendered and colonial practice of claiming ownership over discoveries. The act of 'discovery' involves an act of renaming something under a different logic (e.g., science) but also a manifestation of male anxieties over the need to establish origin (Foster 2016; McClintock 1995). This implies also an erasure of the communities who, for example, produce, oversee, and contribute to knowledge collectively. In the end, the effect of law, through patenting medications, is to cut and uproot the molecule from its context, thus positioning it as a biomedical object without a history under control of the authority of the creator (Foster 2016).

The regulation of safety in herbal medicines has similarly failed to engage on their own terms traditional knowledge systems. This is partly because knowledge in general is inevitably hard to pin down, constantly being shaped and shaping itself anew through people's relations, regulations, contexts, and everyday practices adapting and re-adjusting to new configurations and situations (e.g., Martin et al. 2015). In traditional medicine, this includes, for example, the displacement of practices or products under the pressure to perform in a 'more scientific' way to receive juridical authorisation. While the THMP regime does not specifically exclude other ways of knowing, 'genuine' THMP not only change their formulas but undergo a process of industrial and laboratory inscriptions that render the whole appearance of the product into something else. This 'something else' may or may not resemble a pharmacological product, but it is in any case uprooted from the epistemologies of care and pragmatic testing that do exist and have existed in traditional and herbal medicine histories and practices (Gómez 2013; Langwick 2018). Those who do not comply with such transformations may become both illegitimate in the eyes of the law and regarded as a fake insofar they are often described as irrational and dangerous even when actually for users and knowledge holders there is no doubt as to their 'genuineness'. The role of the law is significant here, both technically and in its ability to participate to broader modes of legitimacy-making (Cloatre 2018). This uncertainty persists in the context of pharmacovigilance, in which the difficulties of the system we described previously are at least in part generated by a lack of engagement with traditional modes of knowing. The next section expands on these issues and argues that uncertainty in traditional herbal medicines is aggravated because regulatory systems rely on herbs being uprooted from the knowledge base they came from.

(G)local plants: dislocated cultures of safety

In the UK and Europe, the case of *kava-kava* (or *piper methysticum*, a crop of the Pacific Islands) brings out to the foreground some of the sticky points in the regulation which remain unsolved, in particular how safety and 'fakeness' are constructed. Following several reports of liver toxicity linked to products with *kava-kava*, the Medicines Control Agency (today the MHRA) prohibited the sale, supply, and importation of this popular herb used to treat anxiety (MHRA 2005). Examining the construction of hepatoxicity through an STS methodology, Baker (2011) argues that the production of knowledge about *kava*'s toxicity is directly related to power and cultural hegemony of biomedicine, including the whole process of research and dissemination of results. In Europe, the plant extract—kavalactones—rose in popularity as an alternative to pharmaceutical industry medicines as an alternative to synthetic drugs against anxiety. However, the German national authorities decided to ban *kava* as a caution and because there were already proven products in the market, such as benzodiazepines.

Although not necessarily safer, there is more knowledge about benzodiazepines from clinical trials. This means the inconclusive evidence about *kava* was an ambiguity exploited both by supporters against the *kava* ban and by regulators who saw the ambiguity as a public health risk. Meanwhile, in Hawaï, where *kava* is used in '*awa*, a traditional drink suppressed during the colonial period and became later a symbol of the resurgence of Hawaiian culture, local pro-*kava* groups' response was to judge how Europeans use their plant incorrectly, namely by transforming it into a pharmacological object. Rather than using all the plant, '*awa* is made with the roots, believed not to contain the hepatotoxic components. They also criticised how the pills contained the cheapest part of the plant (stem peelings), reflecting the hollowing out of the traditional use. In the end, *kava*'s hepatoxicity reflects the failure to factor in safety assessments from the medico-juridical, scientific, and industrial translation, which transform and uproot plants from their socio-historical contexts. It also illustrates a mismatch between the pre-marketing and post-marketing phase, which cuts across the regulatory regime of traditional herbal medicines as we have described previously: while the safety and plausible efficacy of plants in traditional knowledges is recognised in the process of authorisation, safe practices embedded to the tradition itself seem to vanish as reference-points in the post-marketing phase. And, regulatory regimes for sales and distributions may make this more difficult by limiting traditional herbalists' role as knowledge holders and intermediaries between plants and consumers.

To that extent, toxicity is isolated within the laboratory and cut off from the socio-technical assemblages of plants. Contrary to assumptions that growers and producers of herbal medicines are naïve about the toxicity of potent plants, Stacey Langwick argues they interpret toxicity as made up by multiple layers (e.g., embodied, social, political) (Langwick 2018). Yet, the social relationships that surround, produce, and limit toxicity are erased in regulation, as plants are assessed and deployed independently of the networks of knowledge and practice that surround them. As regulators continue to wrestle with the question of which herbs can safely be brought to market, less attention is placed on how connections can be maintained between traditional herbal remedies and traditional knowledge systems. While this is a complicated issue from a regulatory perspective, it is also one without which safety in traditional herbal remedy use can probably not entirely be settled. Similarly, the fear of 'fake' herbal medicines, while certainly justified because of occurrences compromising public health, should not pre-empt a careful engagement with these issues. In fact, clarifying what should count as 'real' traditional herbal medicines, and within which social practices, is a necessary condition to addressing issues of fraudulence.

Conclusions

We have highlighted how the ambivalent location of traditional (herbal) medicines complicates matters related to surveillance of 'fake' herbal medicines. This illustrates both the co-constitution of healing epistemologies and plants, but also the unidirectionality of the constitution of global science, which takes from, but does not engage in, an equitable relation with local knowledges (Pollock 2014). Contemporary regulatory logics, particularly in Europe, demonstrate that both cooperation and conflict co-exist within a hierarchical structure, where laboratory science supersedes traditional knowledge and safety. In the end, herbal medicines are 'unruly objects' that cannot be made to fit into regulatory frameworks without acknowledging the social relationships to which they belong. Both their safety and potential toxicity are deeply entangled in (g)local social, legal, and technological networks. The difficulty for regulators to approach safety and toxicity as rooted in particular systems of knowledge and practice, and the remaining barriers faced by some types of herbal products over others, are also illustrative of persisting epistemological imbalances.

Acknowledgements

This work was supported by the Wellcome Trust grant 200380/Z/15/Z. We would like to thank the editors for their support in the development of this piece.

Note

1 Article 16a (1)(e) of Directive 2004/24/EC of the European Parliament and of the Council of 31 March 2004, amending, as regards traditional herbal medicinal products, Directive 2001/83/EC on the Community code relating to medicinal products for human use.

References

Alliance for Natural Health International (2013) *EU herbal medicines legislation fails again*. Available at: www.anhinternational.org/2013/07/10/eu-herbal-medicines-legislation-fails-again/

Baker J (2011) Tradition and toxicity: evidential cultures in the kava safety debate. *Social Studies of Science* 41(3):361–384

Barnes J (2003) Pharmacovigilance of herbal medicines: a UK perspective. *Drug Safety* 26(12):829–851

BHMA (2019) *Welcome to a new sector of the BHMA, the Herbal Practitioners Suppliers Section (HPSS)*. British Herbal Medicines Association. Available at: https://bhma.info/index.php/hpss/

Biagi M, Pecorari R, Appendino G, Miraldi E, Magnano AR, Governa P, Cettolin G and Giachetti D (2016) Herbal products in Italy: the thin line between phytotherapy, nutrition and parapharmaceuticals: a normative overview of the fastest growing market in Europe. *Pharmaceutical (Basel)* 9(4):E65

Cloatre E (2018) Regulating alternative healing in France, and the problem of 'non-medicine. *Medical Law Review* (online first)

Cocks M and Valerie M (2002) Use of indigenous and indigenised medicines to enhance personal well-being: a South African case study. *Social Science & Medicine* 54:387–397

Corazza O, Martinotti G, Santacroce R, Chillemi E, Di Giannantonio M, Schifano F and Cellek S (2014) Sexual enhancement products for sale online: raising awareness of the psychoactive effects of yohimbine, maca, horny goat weed, and ginkgo biloba. *BioMed Research International*:841798

Corns C and Metcalfe K (2002) Risks associated with herbal slimming remedies. *The Journal of The Royal Society for the Promotion of Health* 122(4):213–219

Derbyshire D (2000) Alternative asthma cures 'could be dangerous'. *The Telegraph*. Oct 24. Available at: www.telegraph.co.uk/news/uknews/1371499/Alternative-asthma-cures-could-be-dangerous.html

Ernst E (1998) Herbs that cure you- or kill you. *The Independent*. Available at: www.independent.co.uk/arts-entertainment/health-herbs-that-can-cure-you-or-kill-you-1183980.html

European Commission (2019) *Pharmacovigilance, public health*. Available at: https://ec.europa.eu/health/human-use/pharmacovigilance_en

European Medicines Agency (2017) *Uptake of the traditional use registration scheme and implementation of the provisions of Directive 2004 / 24 / EC in EU member states, EMA/HMPC/322570/2011 Rev. 5*. London. Available at: www.ema.europa.eu/docs/en_GB/document_library/Report/2011/05/WC500106706.pdf

Evans S (2008) Social science & medicine changing the knowledge base in western herbal medicine. *Social Science & Medicine* 67(12):2098–2106

Fan TP, Deal G, Koo HL, Rees D, Sun H, Chen S, Dou JH, Makarov VG, Pozharitskaya ON, Shikov AN, Kim YS, Huang YT, Chang YS, Jia W, Dias A, Wong VC and Chan K (2012) Future development of global regulations of Chinese herbal products. *Journal of Ethnopharmacology* 140(3):568–586

Foster L (2016) Decolonizing patent law: postcolonial technoscience and indigenous knowledge in South Africa. *Feminist Formations* 28(3):148–173

Gaudillière JP (2002) *Inventer la biomédecine la France, l'Amérique et la production des savoirs du vivant (1945–1965)*. Paris: La Découverte

Gómez PF (2013) The circulation of bodily knowledge in the seventeenth-century black Spanish Caribbean. *Social History of Medicine* 26(3):383–402

Green G, Bradby H, Chan A and Lee M (2006) 'We are not completely westernised': dual medical systems and pathways to health care among Chinese migrant women in England. *Social Science & Medicine* 62:1498–1509

HMAC (2014) *Safety, regulation and herbal medicines: a report prepared by the UK Herbal Medicines Advisory Committee (HMAC) for the Herbal Medicines and Practitioners Working Group (HMPW)*. London. Available at: http://riverfrontmedia.co.uk/EHTPA/HMAC Herbal Safety Report for HMPWG.pdf

House of Lords (2000) *Science and technology: sixth report*. London. Available at: https://publications.parliament.uk/pa/ld199900/ldselect/ldsctech/123/12302.htm

Huntley AL, Coon JT and Ernst E (2005) The safety of herbal medicinal products derived from a systematic review. *Drug Safety* 28(5):387–400

Ijaz N, Boon H, Muzzin L and Welsh S (2016) State risk discourse and the regulatory preservation of traditional medicine knowledge: the case of acupuncture in Ontario, Canada. *Social Science & Medicine* 170:97–105

Jackson E (2012) *Law and the regulation of medicines*. Oxford: Hart Publishing

Kim J (2007) Alternative medicine's encounter with laboratory science: the scientific construction of Korean medicine in a global age. *Social Studies of Science* 37(6):855–880

Langwick SA (2018) A politics of habitability: plants, healing and sovereignty in a toxic world. *Cultural Anthropology* 33(3):415–443

Li W (2002) Botanical drugs: a future for herbal medicines. *A Future for Herbal Medicines* 19(1):117–149

Maclennan E and Pendry BA (2011) The evolution of herbal medicine as an unorthodox branch of British medicine: the role of English legislation from 1914 to the present day. *Journal of Herbal Medicine* 1(2):35–41

Martin A, Myers N and Viseu A (2015) The politics of care in technoscience. *Social Studies of Science* 45(5):625–641

McClintock A (1995) *Imperial leather: race, gender, and sexuality in the colonial contest.* New York: Routledge

McIntyre M (2011) Letters to Editor: regulation of herbal medicines. *The Lancet* 378(9791):569–570

Melvin S (2013) Human medicines: herbal medicines. In Appelbe GE and Wingfield J (eds.) *Dale and Appelbe's pharmacy and medicines law*. Pharmaceutical Press. Available at: https://ecdc.europa.eu/sites/portal/files/media/en/publications/Publications/EU-guidelines-prudent-use-antimicrobials.pdf

MHRA (2005) *Consultation document MLX 319: the medicines for human use (Kava-kava) (Prohibition) Order 2002.* London. Available at: www.mhra.gov.uk/home/groups/commsic/documents/websiteresources/con007682.pdf

NHS England (2017) Items which should not be routinely prescribed in primary care: a Consultation on guidance for CCGs. Available at: www.engage.england.nhs.uk/consultation/items-routinely-prescribed/

Peralta PD, Botija FG and Martin CC (2016) Regulating the risks from traditional herbal medicine resources and herbal supplements in the EU – the borderline products. *European Food and Feed Law Review* 4:274–290

Pickup Z and Hodges C (2002) Recent developments in the regulation of traditional herbal medicines. *International Legal Practitioner* 27(Sept):82–88

Pollock A (2014) Places of pharmaceutical knowledge-making: global health, post-colonial science and hope in South African drug discovery. *Social Studies of Science* 44(6):848–873

Porter R (1999) *The greatest benefit to mankind: a medical history of humanity from antiquity to the present.* London: Fontana Press

Puig M and Bellacasa D (2011) Matters of care in technoscience: assembling neglected things. *Social Studies of Science* 41(1):85–106

Quah SR (2003) Traditional healing systems and the ethos of science. *Social Science & Medicine* 57:1997–2012

RCHM (2019) *FAQ, register of Chinese herbal medicine.* Available at: http://rchm.co.uk/faq/

Ruiz-Poveda O (2015) Regulation of herbal (traditional) medicinal products in the European Union. *Pharmaceutical Regulatory Affairs: Open Access* 4(2):1–5

Saks M (2002) *Orthodox medicine and alternative medicine: politics professionalisation and healthcare.* London: Sage

Scarborough J and Fernandes A (2011) Ancient medicinal use of Aristolochia: birthwort's tradition and toxicity. *Pharmacy in History* 53(1):3–21

Seddon T (2016) Inventing drugs: a genealogy of a regulatory concept. *Journal of Law and Society* 43(3):393–415

Sénat (2018) Sénat Mission d'information sur le développement de l'herboristerie et des plantes médicinales, des filières et métiers d'avenir. "Les plantes médicinales et l'herboristerie: à la croisée de savoirs ancestraux et d'enjeux d'avenir." Rapport d'information de M. Joël LABBÉ, fait au nom de la MI Développement de l'herboristerie n° 727 (2017–2018), 25 septembre 2018. Available at: http://www.senat.fr/notice-rapport/2017/r17-727-notice.html?fbclid=IwAR1gnptJPRRLLx8gSejeY9WXRkbmTi0W4AB4xanoN0M0vBIGK-478NTaHjk

Silano V, Coppens P, Larranaga-Guetaria A, Minghetti P, Roth-Ehrang R (2011) Food & function regulations applicable to plant food supplements and related products in the European Union. *Food and Function* 2:710–719

Urquiza-Haas N (2017) The semiotic fractures of vulnerable bodies: resistance to the gendering of legal subjects. *International Journal for the Semiotics of Law* 30(4):543–562

Virtosu I (2018) The future and prospects of the traditional Chinese medicine on the EU market under new use regulatory framework. *Medicine & Law Review* 37(1):245–276

Wahlberg A (2008) Above and beyond superstition: western herbal medicine and the decriminalizing of placebo. *History of the Human Sciences* 21(1):77–101

Walker D (2015) Report on the regulation of herbal medicines and practitioners. *Department of Health* (Mar). Available at: www.gov.uk/government/uploads/system/uploads/attachment_data/file/417768/Report_on_Regulation_of_Herbal_Medicines_and_Practitioners.pdf

Whitehouse J (2014) Research informing herbal medicine practice. In Brice-Ytsma H and Watkins F (eds.) *Herbal exchanges: in celebration of the national institute of medical herbalists*. London: Strathmore Publishing

WHO (2000) *General guidelines for methodologies on research and evaluation of traditional medicine*. Geneva: World Health Organization

WHO (2002) *Traditional medicine strategy 2002–2005*. Geneva: World Health Organization. Available at: www.wpro.who.int/health_technology/book_who_traditional_medicine_strategy_2002_2005.pdf

WHO (2013) *WHO traditional medicine strategy 2014–2023*. Geneva: World Health Organization. Available at: https://apps.who.int/iris/bitstream/handle/10665/92455/9789241506090_eng.pdf?sequence=

11 Framing of CAM-adjacent health scams in the UK media

An interdisciplinary perspective

Anita Lavorgna and Felicity L. Bishop

Introduction

Complementary and alternative medicine (CAM) is an umbrella term encompassing a broad and heterogeneous range of health care approaches developed outside standard science-based medicine. CAMs are used for health prevention, maintenance, and the treatment of illness (Bishop et al. 2010; EFCAM 2017) mainly outside but sometimes within the structures of conventional health care (Falkenberg et al. 2012).

CAMs have often been at the centre of heated debates and polarised views (Lipman 2002; Segar 2012; Lavorgna and Di Ronco 2017). On the one hand, CAM approaches are promoted as holistic, natural, curative, preventive, enhancing self-healing capacities, and promoting patient-responsibility for health and self-management (EFCAM 2017); they can effectively integrate with allopathic medicine in addressing specific patients' physical, psychological, and spiritual needs (Ernst et al. 2006; Bausell 2007; Bishop et al. 2007; Myers et al. 2012; Deng and Cassileth 2013). On the other hand, CAMs are seen as part of a false dichotomy: to borrow Angell and Kassirer's words, 'there cannot be two kinds of medicine—conventional and alternative. There is only medicine that has been adequately tested and medicine that has not, medicine that works and medicine that may or may not work' (Angell and Kassirer 1998:841). Hence, CAM approaches are accused of being unsupported by scientific evidence and potentially causing harmful side effects (Lerner 1984; Herbert 1986; Sampson 1995; Barrier and Yarett 2012; Cattaneo and Corbellini 2014; Zettler 2015).

Anti-CAM views are often triggered not by Sampson legitimate CAMs (for instance, in the UK, those recognised by the Complementary and Natural Healthcare Council) but by countless outright fraudulent pseudoscientific practices (such as bogus anti-cancer treatments and other 'quackeries') that self-denominate as 'CAM' and that are, or are likely to be, seriously harmful for the patient (hereafter 'CAM-adjacent health scams'). Think of the infamous case of Ryke Geerd Hamer, a German theologian and a former doctor promoting 'alternative' anti-cancer treatment, convicted by several courts for the death of a number of his patients (D'Amato 2010 and Chapter 12; Lavorgna and Di Ronco 2017). In line with existing research (Lavorgna and

Di Ronco 2018), the categorisation of certain CAMs as scams in this study will depend on the shifting balance between benefits (health, quality of life, psychological, spiritual) and harms to people (health, emotional and psychological, financial).

As CAMs are broadly used in western countries, spurred by general societal changes such as consumer movements and postmodernism (Coulter and Willis 2004), it is not surprising that media have been reporting on them. Media representations of CAMs are important because the perceptions people have of medical treatments and approaches, including CAMs, can be strongly influenced by the media: previous research highlights how the media helps to disseminate information for consumers considering using CAMs, and that such information, alongside personal recommendations and word of mouth, is influential in consumers' decision-making (Evans et al. 2007; Weeks and Strudsholm 2008; Nissen et al. 2013). For instance, a study of the behaviour of participants of a major Italian-speaking online forum promoting alternative medical treatments (Lavorgna and Di Ronco 2017) showed that forum members placed unlimited trust in a few fake experts (proved to be fraudulent by way of judicial decisions) and suggested that the media may have conveyed ambiguous messages on their potentially dangerous treatments. A follow-up study (Lavorgna and Di Ronco 2018) furthered this path of inquiry by analysing media representations of CAMs in Italy. The authors analysed how the two most-read Italian national generalist newspapers and Italian press news have represented CAMs over time, confirming a great deal of confusion in the press as to what CAMs are, with articles often failing to provide a useful distinction between CAMs and CAM-adjacent health scams. Journalists were often muddling up very different CAM approaches, disregarding the scientific evidence on the effectiveness (or lack of effectiveness) of different treatments. Also, the study showed how Italian media generally failed to frame cases of CAM-adjacent health scams as 'frauds', hence failing to fully recognise the criminal and social harms brought about by them. This is in line with the results of an earlier scoping review looking at research related to CAMs and the mass media carried out in the 1990s and early 2000s, where it was shown that most media do not articulate differences in the treatments and fail to report many issues related to risk and safety (Weeks and Strudsholm 2008).

Media sources, however, might also have the potential to help support informed decision-making and reduce risky behaviours such as consulting unqualified practitioners or falling victim to outright fraudsters and being misled into adopting potentially harmful practices. This would be particularly important in the context of a confusing and inconsistent regulatory situation that can be difficult for consumers to navigate. For example, patients seeking acupuncture in the UK may consult a medical doctor, subject to statutory regulation by the General Medical Council, who might have undertaken a weekend course in acupuncture, or a traditional acupuncturist who might have undertaken a three-year full-time degree but who is not subject to statutory regulation.

This chapter presents a media framing analysis of CAM-adjacent health scams in the UK. By incorporating criminological and psychological perspectives, this study considers both the nature of the health scams as represented in the press news and how their specific framing might inform different types of responses among the readers. The ultimate aim is to better understand how UK news might have shaped public understanding of CAM-adjacent health scams in the UK.

Methodology

Data collection

This study focuses on newspaper articles published in the UK between 1 January 2006 and 31 December 2016. The dates were chosen to capture articles over a period sufficient to consider possible changes over time. In particular, we decided to start our analysis in January 2006, the year of the *Fraud Act* ('An Act to make provision for, and in connection with, criminal liability for fraud and obtaining services dishonestly'), which gives a statutory definition of the criminal offence of fraud (by false representation; by failing to disclose information; by abuse of position). We expected that the new Act might have given a new legal framework to deal with cases of CAM-adjacent health scams (and possibly increase media and public attention to the issue).

Articles were extracted from the database *LexisNexis Academic*, which provides full text access to press news and allows searches by period, language, and type of source. Trying to keep the search as comprehensive as possible, the following syntaxes were chosen for the keyword searches: 'scam AND health AND medicine' (anywhere in the text, 711 results); 'quack* AND health' (anywhere in the text, 1,671 results); '(alternative medicine) AND (death OR fraud OR scam OR con OR harm)' (in headline and lead paragraphs, 118 results); 'advert* AND (herbal OR medicine)' (in headline and lead paragraphs, 213 results). The search was entered based on the following criteria: timeframe (01/01/2006–31/12/2016) and type of source (UK publication). Duplicate options were automatically excluded 'if high similarity' was to be found. After these preliminary keyword searches, articles were manually sorted out to exclude those non-relevant for the scope of this study (e.g., articles focusing on counterfeited pharmaceuticals; articles on generic 'slimming pills' without any reference to CAMs or frauds; articles dismissive of CAMs in general, including what we categorised as 'beneficial CAMs' for the scope of our study; articles on non-UK cases) and to further eliminate duplicates. A total of 126 press items were identified as relevant and included in the analysis.

As already underlined by Weaver and Bimber (2008), among others, news aggregation databases such as *LexisNexis* have important limitations, which might limit the accuracy of a study looking at the news distribution of a particular subject. In fact, they do not necessarily constitute archives of the whole content of news appearing because of the exclusion of major wire services and major newspapers. Nonetheless, *LexisNexis Academic* was chosen as a proper news aggregator for this exploratory analysis because of its powerful search capability and extensive coverage (Ryan and Simon 2013).

Data analysis

We conceptualised our data in two distinct ways. First, from a criminological perspective, news articles were considered as a representation of cases of CAM-adjacent health scams. From this perspective, the analytic focus was on describing the nature of the health scams as represented in the articles. In particular, we were interested in the specific cases reported, when and where they occurred, the central actors (those who were given voice and the fake CAM expert accused of perpetrating the scams), and the nature of the interventions and patient groups targeted. Second, from a psychological perspective, news articles were considered as potentially shaping readers' views of CAM-adjacent health scams and CAM more broadly. From this perspective, the analytic focus was on considering how CAM scams were constructed in the articles and the ways in which this might encourage or discourage different responses among readers. Specifically, attention was paid to the linguistic resources used to frame stories on CAM scams, as these are seen as having a role in shaping the discursive setting within which readers talk, think, and behave in relation to this topic. To integrate these two perspectives into a coherent analysis, we drew on media framing analysis (Giles and Shaw 2009; Giles et al. 2009; Shaw and Giles 2009).

Media framing analysis focuses on six analytic concepts: the story (also known as the 'news peg'), the characters, reader identification, narrative structure, language categories, and generalisation (Giles and Shaw 2009). We adapted these concepts for our analysis as follows. *Identifying the story* involved ascertaining and describing the specific CAM-adjacent health scam, or case, that had triggered the article. We were interested in the scam itself (i.e., what intervention was being offered for what condition) and when and where the cases occurred. Identifying the *cast of characters* involved identifying individual agents mentioned in the article, including those accused of perpetrating the scams, targets or victims of the scam, and people given voice to comment. The cast of characters was then examined in the context of the article as a whole to identify which character (if any) readers were being invited to identify with. An analysis of *narrative structure and language* focused on the types of articles published and how language was used to construct CAM-adjacent health scams; particular attention was paid to terminology, rhetorical devices (e.g., metaphor), and categories. *Generalisation* involves considering the broader context of the frames and findings; in this study, this was operationalised by comparing the findings to those identified in the previous study of media representations of similar scams in Italy (Lavorgna and Di Ronco 2018). Finally, these elements were brought together to identify the dominant overarching frames used to present CAM-adjacent scams to readers and consider how they might encourage or discourage different responses.

The process of developing a media framing analysis involves working closely with the raw data and gradually building up an understanding of the frames. NVivo 11, a data analysis software package that allows one to manage and arrange unstructured information, was used to systematically organise and analyse the data sampled from the documents. Low-level codes were developed in accordance with the first five analytic concepts described in the previous paragraph (the story, the characters, reader identification, narrative structure, and language categories). For example, a group of codes was developed to describe the people involved in the stories (the 'cast of characters'), and these codes were used to code all mentions of people throughout the data corpus. In order to facilitate comparative analysis, we utilised codes developed by Lavorgna and Di Ronco (2018) whenever possible, adding new codes when needed based on a close reading of the articles to reflect specific features of UK media reporting and to incorporate elements of media framing analysis not used in the Italian study. Low-level codes were then compared and revisited within the context of the articles as a whole, in order to identify the overarching frames. Besides assisting us with qualitative analysis, NVivo allowed us to count the number of times each code was used across the sampled articles. An audit trail, incorporating definitions of codes, was maintained throughout, and the two authors worked collaboratively on data coding and interpretation.

Please note that in our analysis and discussion we are not providing the full names of the those involved in the CAM-adjacent health scams, because in some cases the media news refers to an open investigation and also because we want to avoid advertising (allegedly fraudulent) practitioners.

Results and discussion

Identifying the story

The trigger

The vast majority of the press news appears to have been triggered by a variety of causes such as the arrest or the recent speech of a fake CAM specialist, a warning issued by the police, or an interview with a CAM (or anti-CAM) expert. Only in seven cases (out of 126) was the story triggered by a specific case involving an identified patient.

CAM-adjacent interventions at the heart of the scams

Among the CAM techniques most often referred to in the stories on scams were those linked to nutritional vitamins and supplements (28), naturopathy (18), faith healing (15), homeopathy (14), Chinese traditional medicine (13), the use of 'special' untested machineries (11), magnetic bioenergetics therapy (7), the use of untested pharmaceuticals and medical procedures (7), bleach treatment (6), physical manipulation (6), and detox practices (5). Other interventions (including crystal therapy, the use of special oils, iridology, hypnosis, and many more) are referred to 22 items (less than 3 references each). Interestingly, the news often referred to CAMs in general, without specifying a specific intervention (15). Notably, CAM-adjacent scam interventions were explicitly coupled with stopping conventional treatments in 10 cases.

The setting of the stories: 'when' and 'where'

In line with the Italian results, the number of articles published around the topic of CAM-adjacent health scams does not appear to have significantly changed over time; no specific trend (increasing or decreasing number of news articles) could be identified. However, it was possible to observe a concentration of news in specific geographical areas—namely Wales (15 references), the London area (11), the South East (10), and the East Midlands (8). The Italian media analysis also identified geographical patterning. In comparison to the Italian results, however, the UK news articles do not seem to concentrate on specific cities, partially contradicting the suggestion that social networks developed in a specific territory could have a role in explaining the concentration of CAM-adjacent health scams. Further comparative research, also analysing specifically local press, could help in clarifying the geographical distribution of CAM-adjacent health scams. Finally, many news articles (44) presented an international element (e.g., the CAM product was imported from abroad).

Cast of characters and reader identification

The individual agents involved in the stories were the victims, those accused of perpetrating the scams, and those who were given a 'voice' with whom the reader was invited to identify, such as qualified experts.

The victims

We identified seven different cases where the news focused on a specific and clearly identifiable patient (fraud victim) who was severely harmed by CAM-adjacent health scams. These are the cases of N (child, male) (3); SMC (58, male, actor) (2); LW (male, international student); AB (80, male, disabled) (2); MB (57, female) (1); BJ (child, male) (1); DP (52, female) (1). Overall, UK media tend to give limited attention to specific cases, while in Italy many newspapers were covering the same cases, often giving rise to nation-wide debates. In line with the Italian analysis, statements in the news themselves suggest that the real number of cases of CAM-adjacent health scams is significantly higher: the dark number of cases (and media underreporting) is not surprising and in line with criminological analysis on frauds (Tunley 2014). Consider for instance: 'The UK's Office of Fair Trading says that every year hundreds of thousands of consumers buy scam miracle cures for conditions such as weight loss, baldness and impotence', *Daily Mirror*, 27 March 2015; '[the victim] found himself on a 'sucker's list which grew over a period of 22 years . . . The UK charity Think Jessica believes this is "the tip of the iceberg"', *Daily Mirror*, 2 October 2015).

Scams were most frequently described as targeting people with cancer (61), in line with the Italian results. This confirms how many CAM-adjacent health scams are directed at people made potentially vulnerable by serious and often terminal serious illness. Other stories addressed: health issues in general with no reference to a specific disease (16); HIV (15); so-called lifestyle problems such as weight loss, baldness, and impotence (15); arthritis (10); beauty and wellbeing in general (7); autism (in the context of the so-called vaccine conspiracy) (6); chronic fatigue syndrome (6); multiple sclerosis, Parkinson's disease, motor neuron disease, etc. (6); infertility (5); malaria (3); mental health (3); minor health issues (such as fever and a minor injury) (3); cornea erosion (1); and phlebitis (1). Interestingly enough, there was also one case of *ndoki* (a form of demonic possession) and two on the use of homeopathic medicines to 'cure' homosexuality. Again in line with the Italian results, our UK study shows the extreme heterogeneity of people, ranging from seriously ill patients to the 'worried well', who were described as the victims of CAM-adjacent health scams in the media. In the UK (contrary to in Italy), however, specific attention was drawn to the severe harms (physical, emotional, and financial) suffered by the victims as a consequence of the scams (86), which is encouraging regarding the potential role of the media in alerting the public to the dangers of CAM-adjacent health scams.

The perpetrators

UK media, contrary to the Italian ones, did not cluster their attention towards some major fake health 'experts' advocating dangerous (and often international) CAM-adjacent health scams. While in the Italian media, for instance, the relative majority of news on quackeries referred to the infamous Rykw Geerd Hamer (the originator of the Germanic New Medicine, see D'Amato 2010 and Chapter 12), in the UK an overwhelming majority of news focused on cases with local impact and small-scale reach. Even in the case of Dr SH, whose approach was clearly Hamerian and who—as he was given voice in the article—made references to Simoncini (another sadly known controversial 'expert', active in several countries, promoting an alternative dangerous anti-cancer treatment) (Di Grazia 2015; Lavorgna and Di Ronco 2017), the media news did not take the chance to explain to the readers the broader context and the dangers of the approach at the basis of Dr SH's therapies. Apart from the case of the Gs, a couple at the centre of a health fraud resulting in a sexual assault covered by some media (10 references), no other perpetrator surpassed the three references. In line with the Italian results, most named perpetrators are men and come from different backgrounds: besides doctors (or former doctors) are those with no experience in the medical sector and spiritual healers (or self-named 'archbishops'). Furthermore, some stories also suggested the significant involvement of people operating in the traditional healthcare system in CAM-adjacent scams (e.g., pharmacists or nurses facilitating the initial contact between the victim and the scammer), emphasising once more the importance of further research into the role and the responsibilities of these facilitators.

Many articles described how fraudsters advertised their interventions and attempted to gain their victims' trust (64). The most common such methods involved word of mouth (especially for many dangerous anti-cancer scams, where the victim is often referred to the practitioner via a common acquaintance), phone calls (especially for scams targeting older adults, trying to sell them 'natural' health products), and leaflets dropped through letterboxes or left on car windscreens. Online advertisement is also increasingly used (via dedicated websites, e-shops, chats, and other social media). Especially when the victims are approached via phone calls, the scammer first pretends to build up a rapport with them and then pressurises them to buy expensive items. When the relationship is built in person, the perpetrator is always presented as a trustworthy and reliable expert. Furthermore, perpetrators often target their victims among specific social groups (e.g., via online forums), directing their efforts in an effective way. For instance, similar to the Italian cases, many CAM-adjacent health scammers are appealing to those who had chosen a specific 'lifestyle' (14 references) (e.g., 'Millions of people have made alternative health a lifestyle choice', *The Bristol Post*, 17 March 2008).

Voice and reader identification

The group most often given a voice was qualified experts (such as doctors, researchers, and notorious debunkers) (44), followed by people with a vested interest in CAM (practitioners, CAM-related business companies, and their attorneys—27 references in total). Interestingly, when voice was given to the latter group, legitimate CAM approaches were at times presented in a positive light and in three extreme cases incorporated proactive advertisements of CAM businesses or products. In addition, politicians and administrative authorities (22) were at times quoted, mostly to warn their constituency about the dangers of CAM-adjacent scams. The UK media, compared to the Italian media, tended to give more 'voice' to criminal justice actors such as public prosecutors (16) and patients/victims (or one of their friends or family members, or their attorneys—16 references in total), and less to famous people (e.g., actors, bloggers, etc., without a specific medical expertise), whose voices appear only in 6 news articles. This difference, however, could be explained by the differences in the case selection: the Italian analysis focused on CAM representations in general, even if the focus of the research was on fraudulent activities; our UK study looks at CAM-adjacent health scams only. Very little voice was given to the general public (at times referred to as potential victims, should the scam not be identified—7 references), charities (such as anti-fraud charities lacking a specific expertise on CAM-adjacent health scams) (4), religious authorities (3), CAM associations (the British Homeopathic Association, the Society of Homeopaths, and the Prince's Foundation for Integrated Health—3 references in total), the medical associations and ethics committee (2), and former CAM practitioners (1 reference only). Contrary to the Italian results, in the UK no voice was given to patients' associations.

The dominance of the voice of qualified experts and the relative paucity of victims' voices suggests that it is with the experts that readers were typically invited to identify. In other words, readers were invited to take a position as a rational actor, encouraged to see fraudulent claims for what they are and not be taken in or victimised by them. Further support for this interpretation comes from the presence, in 17 articles, of explicit advice to readers on how to behave should they encounter CAM-adjacent health scams. This advice not only encourages the reader not to be taken in but also enlists them in the surveillance and policing of scams. Consider, for instance: 'If you have concerns, consumers can contact the Citizens Advice Consumer Service on 03454 040506', *Eastwood & Kimberley Advertiser*, 7 July 2016; 'Anyone who receives potentially fraudulent mail should report it to the Royal Mail help line on 03456 113413 or emailscam.mail@royalmail.com', *Mirror*, 2 October 2015.

Narrative structure and language

The articles were most commonly presented as news stories (42 references), although it was not possible to identify all article types from the *LexisNexis* record. Other common categories were features (19), columns/opinions (10), and life/style, society, consumer affairs, or culture (13) articles. There were also seven articles in health or medicine sections, two in the sport section, and one front page piece.

The language used to describe CAM-adjacent scams drew on discourses of science, religion, nature, business, and crime. Scams were constructed as the antithesis of scientific medicine, as involving unproven interventions which lacked any evidence to support their claims of being able to provide relief, to heal, to cure, or to have other such beneficial effects (for example, 'It seems a depressing reality that while desperate people exist to exploit, scientific reality will often be ignored and dubious fictions substituted in its stead', *The Guardian*, 15 July 2015).

Victims of scams were described as believing, trusting, or having faith in a convincing perpetrator, and feeling, thinking, or hoping they might benefit from a 'miracle' cure, remedy, therapy, or treatment. Stark contrasts were drawn with scientific medicine, constructed as evidence-based with known benefits proven in rigorous clinical trials conducted by scientists/researchers and interpreted by highly qualified experts. For example,

> I called Dr D to find out if she would agree to prescribe me a drug called laetrile Z sometimes known as amygdalin, or Vitamin B17 Z derived from apricot kernels. Advocates of the treatment believe it can shrink cancerous tumours, despite numerous scientific trials proving this to be false. The chemical also converts to cyanide in the body, and has been responsible for the deaths of a number of cancer patients.
>
> (*Mail on Sunday*, 3 October 2010)

According to the articles, scam interventions themselves had often been marketed as more natural or traditional alternatives to mainstream (chemical, harmful, toxic) medicine, drawing on the common, mistaken, assumption that natural equals safe and using associated terms such as detoxification. In some articles, these claims were compared with the lack of effects or even harmful (sometimes toxic) effects that the interventions could actually have.

> AH, 50, imported the herbal remedy, which he described as a natural alternative to traditional treatments including chemotherapy. He claimed he himself was in remission from cancer after taking it. . . . He charged £250 for 100 tablets which he described as 'nature's miraculous alternative' and an 'excellent supplement or logical alternative to chemotherapy, to shrink tumours'.
>
> (*Manchester Evening News*, 7 September 2012)

Scams were sometimes described primarily in business or economic terms, with perpetrators charging people often extortionate amounts of money for unproven products or processes and thus causing financial harm to their victims. For example:

> Desperate to walk again, AB gave a staggering £300 a week to fake companies all over the world who claimed they could treat his health problems. After being lured in by the prospect of cash bonuses which he hoped would pay for private healthcare, his name was added to a so-called suckers' list of people likely to respond to appeals.
>
> (*Daily Mail*, 3 October 2015)

Such scammers were portrayed as con artists, out for financial gain, working within an industry that also at times included more legitimate businesses such as well-known health shops. As previous research suggested that many victims and/or supporters of dangerous quackeries are seduced by them as they are seen in opposition to the 'greedy big-Pharma' (Lavorgna and Di Ronco 2017), this type of narrative might prove useful to discourage potential victims from undertaking harmful treatments.

Finally, a small number of particularly serious scams were described as illegal criminal acts of frauds (or other offences including indecent assault), perpetrated on innocent and often vulnerable victims by alleged or accused suspects and criminals who were subsequently investigated and caught by police or trading standards and sentenced and/or jailed by the judiciary.

Overarching frames and their potential impact on readers

After analysing the individual components of the frames as noted previously (story, the characters, reader identification, narrative structure, and language categories), these elements were then brought together to identify the dominant overarching frames used to present CAM-adjacent scams to readers and consider how they might encourage or discourage different responses. Three such frames were identified and are described in the next sections: a legal frame, an economic frame, and a medical frame.

A legal frame

This frame employs a criminal justice and a regulatory narrative. In the criminal justice version, scams are perpetrated by suspects, criminals, and/or defendants, they have victims (and potential victims) or complainants, and must be stopped and punished by the judiciary. For example, a number of articles reported on the case of RG and LG who were convicted and jailed at Swansea Crown Court: 'A PENSIONER was jailed for eight years today after molesting a Gwent woman under the guise of offering alternative medicine' (*South Wales Argus*, 11 April 2012, emphasis in the original). In the regulatory version, scams are perpetrated by unregulated individuals, they have victims (and potential victims) or complainants, and need to be prevented by regulators. In both forms of the legal frame, readers were often explicitly encouraged to contact officials to report suspicious activity: contact details for the police, crime-stoppers, trading standards, and (less often) council officials were commonly provided at the end of articles. Consider, for instance, the following extract:

> Trading standards manager RR has said: 'This type of scam preys on the most vulnerable people and will offer to cure diseases or to mend broken relationships. Anyone with health problems should visit their GP and we would be very worried about people relying on a faith healer instead of proper medical care. There are genuine organisations out there for people who need help with their health or any other aspects of their lives'. Information can be passed to Leicestershire Police on 101 or Crimestoppers, which is anonymous, on 0800 555111.
>
> (*Leicester Mercury*, 7 November 2015)

An economic frame

This frame brings attention to scams as a form of business: perpetrators are peddlers and con artists who are motivated by profit and victims stand to lose (sometimes considerable amounts of) money. There is an associated industry which supports the scams, manufacturing products that are then advertised and marketed (making baseless claims) and sold to consumers. This frame can also encompass stories that mention well-known brands and shops which sell products with what are described as unproven, but claimed, benefits. The victims of scams are 'vulnerable' consumers, who may be made vulnerable by virtue of their age (older adults), circumstance (e.g., recently widowed, living alone), and/or health issues (e.g., arthritis, pain, fatigue). The economic frame focuses on the financial benefits (for perpetrators) and financial costs (for victims), encouraging the reader to see the scam interventions as fraudulent, fake, or bogus products and the perpetrators as profiteers rather than health care providers. For example, *The Eastwood Advertiser* (7 July 2016) under the headline 'scammers target elderly' began an article as follows:

> Vulnerable people are being targeted by high pressure sales calls to buy nutritional supplements and painkilling remedies on the telephone—according to the council. As part of national Scams Awareness Month, Nottinghamshire County Council's Trading Standards team has revealed it is supporting a number of vulnerable people who have bought nutritional supplements following sales calls they have taken out of the blue. They are concerned people are buying goods which may not offer any health or wellbeing benefits.

The article went on to provide examples of recent cases, including:

> One resident who agreed to buy 30 tubes of pain relieving cream for joints which could be bought over the counter for a fraction of the £31 per tube he was charged. [And] Someone who was sold a huge amount of different products including 20 packets of pomegranate supplements for £500.

A medical frame

This frame emphasises the medical context and consequences of the scams and draws heavily on discourses of science and evidence-based medicine. Scientists, doctors, and other expert debunkers are given voice and draw clear distinctions between western scientific medicine and the scam products or processes. However, they may also draw parallels between the scam and (arguably legitimate) forms of CAM, for instance by equating them to acupuncture or herbal medicine. Articles in this frame focus on how the intervention cannot do what it claims to do, the lack of evidence to support the claims made, and the potential for harmful effects on patient-victims' health. The plight of the victim is often vividly described as a fight for survival at all costs, a patient who is taken advantage of by fake or disgraced doctors, self-proclaimed healers, and other perpetrators. Consider for instance the following example:

> He is a prime example of the new breed of complementary and alternative practitioners. Gone are the beads-and-incense brigade peddling herbs and crystals. Today's snake-oil salesmen are slick, suited and often medically qualified and all too willing to cash in on the desperation of vulnerable patients. From private clinics in prestigious addresses, they bamboozle patients with pseudo-science while pushing extortionately expensive yet ultimately useless and even dangerous treatments. What Dr T . . . does should be a criminal offence. The GMC insists that its sanctions are 'not to

> punish . . . but to protect patients'. Until tougher measures are brought in, disciplining the likes of him is little more than a token gesture.
>
> (*Mail on Sunday*, 3 October 2010)

The medical frame appears the most likely to present potential problems, for both CAM professionals and their patients. This is because of the way in which parallels are drawn between CAM-adjacent scams and legitimate CAMs (or distinctions between the two are even obscured, as in the *Mail on Sunday* excerpt), and the overly simplistic contrasts that are drawn between scientific medicine and all other interventions. This may deter some consumers from seeking legitimate CAMs. It may also inadvertently put some consumers at risk of scams, if they react to an inappropriately strong anti-CAM message by ignoring (or rejecting) the important anti-fraud messages.

In line with the findings of the Italian study, journalists tended to muddle up very different CAM approaches when reporting on CAM-related issues, disregarding not only the scientific evidence on the effectiveness of different treatments but also the diverse levels of harms at stake. In order to overcome this confusion, journalists dealing with health-related issues should receive ad hoc training and, if needed, experts presenting evidence-based accounts on sensitive topics should be more involved in mainstream media to help the general public to develop informed opinions (Lavorgna and Di Ronco 2018).

Concluding remarks

Our focus in this chapter has been on media framing of CAM-adjacent health scams. The analysis has shown that, despite the fact that CAM-adjacent health scams are likely to be a large-scale—even if very underreported—issue in the UK, the attention they receive in the mainstream media is still limited and their representation is often superficial. Particularly, we have seen how UK media use legal, economic, and medical frames when reporting on CAM-adjacent health scams. Aspects of these frames can be confusing, in-depth journalistic analyses are missing, and instances of scams are generally covered as isolated cases, without contextualising them within the broader issue of fraudulent pseudoscientific practices. The results also suggest that there might be a geographical patterning in cases of CAM-adjacent health scams and that people operating in the official healthcare system are sometimes involved in some of these scams, two observations deserving further investigation.

We have not performed a comparative analysis to determine the extent and ways in which such framing is similar to or different from the framing of health scams in general, which would have exceeded the scope of this study. Unfortunately, to the authors' knowledge, at the moment there are no existing studies that would allow us to draw a comparison on this point. We suggest that CAM provides one set of discourses (e.g., discourses around nature and holism) that scam perpetrators can draw on in order to target a particular audience, and this suggests that CAM-adjacent scams and their reporting may share many features with mainstream health scams; however, this speculation goes beyond the analysis presented here and requires further study.

Overall the UK media, compared to the Italian one, succeed in their legal and economic frames in demonstrating more attention to the protection of vulnerable customers (for instance, proving them with the contact details of the authorities to denounce the wrong suffered) and to the financial losses they might suffer (by insisting on the scammers' greed). These are certainly good practices that could be used more consistently in UK media and possibly expanded abroad. The medical frame, by contrast, remains problematic: in line with previous media analyses (Weeks and Strudsholm 2008; Lavorgna and Di Ronco 2018), our study shows that media understanding and framing of CAM-adjacent health scams is potentially confounding for readers. This may lead to misunderstandings that could on the one hand deter people from seeking legitimate CAM and on the other hand put people at risk from scams. Better dissemination of scientific research via mainstream media and improved outreach media could have an important impact in preventing CAM-adjacent health scams.

Acknowledgements

We would like to thank the late Laura Little and Daniel Scanlan for their precious contribution in the data collection for this study. This study is part of the project 'Hush the quacks. Exploring health fraud scams in the UK', funded by the Strategic Interdisciplinary Research Development Fund, Faculty of Social Sciences, University of Southampton.

References

Angell M and Kassirer JP (1998) Alternative medicine: the risks of untested and unregulated remedies. *New England Journal of Medicine* 339(12):839–341

Barrier CR and Yarett IR (2012) Cancer quackery: the persistent popularity of useless, irrational 'alternative' treatments. *Oncology* 26(8):754–758

Bausell RB (2007) *Snake oil science: the truth about complementary and alternative medicine.* Oxford: Oxford University Press

Bishop FL, Yardley L and Lewith GT (2007) A systematic review of beliefs involved in the use of complementary and alternative medicine. *Journal of Health Psychology* 12(6):851–867

Bishop FL, Yardley L and Lewith GT (2010) Why consumers maintain complementary and alternative medicine use: a qualitative study. *The Journal of Alternative and Complementary Medicine* 16(2):175–182

Cattaneo E and Corbellini G (2014) Taking a stand against pseudoscience. *Nature* 510:333–335

Coulter I and Willis E (2004) The rise of complementary and alternative medicine: a sociological perspective. *Medical Journal of Australia* 180(11):587–589

D'Amato I (2010) Dossier Hamer. Una valutazione critica basata sui documenti. Available at: www.dossierhamer.it/index.html

Deng G and Cassileth B (2013) Complementary or alternative medicine in cancer care: myths and realities. *Nature Reviews Clinical Oncology* 10(11):656–664

Di Grazia S (2015) La cura Simoncini: una bufala pericolosa. *MedBunker.* Available at: http://medbunker.blogspot.co.uk/p/la-cura-simoncini-non-cura-nessuno.html

EFCAM (2017) European federation for alternative and complementary medicine. Available at: www.efcam.eu/ (18 Nov 2018)

Ernst E, Pittler MH and Wider B (2006) *The desktop guide to complementary and alternative medicine: an evidence-based approach*. London: Mosby

Evans M, Shaw A, Thompson EA, Falk S, Turton P, Thompson T and Sharp D (2007) Decisions to use complementary and alternative medicine (CAM) by male cancer patients: information-seeking roles and types of evidence used. *BMC Complementary and Alternative Medicine* 7(25)

Falkenberg T, Lewith G, Roberti di Sarsina P, von Ammon K, Santos-Rey K, Hök J, Frei-Erb M, Vas J, Saller R, Uehleke B (2012) Towards a pan-European definition of complementary and alternative medicine: a realistic ambition? *Forsch Komplementmed* 19(2):6–8

Giles D and Shaw RL (2009) The psychology of news influence and the development of media framing analysis. *Social and Personality Psychology Compass* 3:375–393

Giles D, Shaw RL and Morgan W (2009) Representations of voluntary childlessness in the UK press, 1990–2008. *Journal of Health Psychology* 14:1218–1228

Herbert V (1986) Unproven (questionable) dietary and nutritional methods in cancer prevention and treatment. *Cancer* 58(S8):1930–1941

Lavorgna A and Di Ronco (2017) Fraud victims or unwary accomplices? An exploratory study of online communities supporting quack medicine. In van Duyne PC, Harvey J, Antonopoulos GA and von Lampe K (eds.) *The many faces of crime for profit and way of tackling it*. Oisterwijk, NL: Wolf Legal Publishers

Lavorgna A and Di Ronco A (2018) Media representations of complementary and alternative medicine in the Italian press: a criminological perspective. *European Journal of Criminology* 15(4):421–441

Lerner IJ (1984) The whys of cancer quackery. *Cancer* 53:815–819

Lipman AG (2002) The polarised debate over complementary and alternative medicine. *Journal of Pain & Palliative Care Pharmacotherapy* 16(4):79–84

Myers SP, Xue CC, Cohen MM, Phelps KL and Lewith GT (2012) Editorial: the legitimacy of academic complementary medicine. *Medical Journal of Australia* 197(2):69–70

Nissen N, Johannessen H, Schunder-Tatzber S, Lazarus A and Weinenhammer W (2013) Citizens' need and attitudes towards CAM. CAMbrella project. Available at: www.cam-europe.eu/dms/files/CAMbrella_Reports/CAMbrella-WP3 final.pdf

Ryan D and Simon J (2013) Broadcast news transcripts in academic news databases. Centre for Research Libraries. Available at: www.crl.edu/sites/default/files/d6/images/tg/Broadcast%20Transcripts% 20Review%202013%20final.pdf

Sampson W (1995) Antiscience trends in the rise of the 'alternative medicine' movement. *Annals of the New York Academy of Sciences* 775(1):188–197

Segar J (2012) Complementary and alternative medicine: exploring the gap between evidence and usage. *Health* 16(4):366–381

Shaw RL and Giles DC (2009) Motherhood on ice? A media framing analysis of older mothers in the UK news. *Psychology & Health* 24:221–236

Tunley M (2014) *Mandating the measurement of fraud: legislating against loss*. London: Palgrave Macmillan

Weaver DA and Bimber B (2008) Finding news stories: a comparison of searches using LexisNexis and Google News. *Journalism and Mass Communication Quarterly* 85(3):515–530

Weeks LC and Strudsholm T (2008) A scoping review of research on complementary and alternative medicine (CAM) and the mass media: looking back, moving forward. *BMC Complementary and Alternative Medicine* 8(43):1–9

Zettler PJ (2015) Compassionate use of experimental therapies: who should decide? *EMBO Molecular Medicine: Perspectives* 7(10):1248–1250

12 Dossier Hamer

The role of investigative journalism in exposing pseudomedicine

Ilario D'Amato

Introduction

In October 1981, the German physician Ryke Geerd Hamer announced on Bavarian and Italian public broadcasting services that he had discovered a 'new medicine'—the so-called Germanic New Medicine (hereafter, GNM)—which he claimed was able to cure 98% of patients suffering from all kinds of diseases (Sigmaringen's Administrative Court 2005). Hamer's theory is based on 'Five Biological Laws of Nature', including the belief that 'so-called diseases as we have understood them until now do not exist. Rather, they are Meaningful Special Biological Programs of Nature' (Hamer 2005:2). According to Hamer, diseases are caused by 'biological conflicts' and do not have to be treated through therapies but must 'be left to run their course because they always have a biological purpose' (Hamer 2005:2). In his opinion, chemotherapy and morphine are instruments of mass murder, a 'holocaust' organised by the Jewish community to kill non-Jewish people (Hamer 2010). Hamer and his supporters claim GNM is hindered by the Jewish community and Big Pharma.

Hamer's biography, as described on his own website and those of his supporters, contrasts starkly with the official documents available and falsely depicts him as a genius hunted down by the establishment. In reality, Hamer lost his licence to practice medicine in 1986 for medical malpractice after treating many patients resulting in irreversible damage or death. However, he continued to practice GNM, and for that was sentenced for illegal practice of medicine, negligence towards a person in danger, libel, and fraud in Germany, Austria, France, and Spain (Administrative Court of Frankfurt Am Main 2003). From journalistic accounts and trial documents, we know that he is responsible for the deaths of more than 140 people (Deckers 2008). In 2007, Hamer fled to Norway to escape a German warrant for his anti-Semitic crimes (Camilletti 2007). From there, he continued to promote his ideas until his death in July 2017 (Lofstad 2017).

By drawing on my journalistic enquiry into Ryke Geerd Hamer's GNM and my efforts to educate the public about its dangers, in this chapter I argue that factual debunking alone cannot counter the appeal of pseudomedicine. A different approach is required.

Exposing Hamer's dangerous myths

2007–2011: my journalistic enquiry and its early dissemination

I first encountered Hamer's GNM in 2007, through an online forum: MeetUp. Two years before, Beppe Grillo—an Italian comedian and political activist—urged the many followers of his blog to 'meet up, discuss issues, step forward, see one another in person' (Grillo 2005). The tool chosen for this civic grassroots movement was the MeetUp platform, which was divided into local groups and had also a national forum. I was among the first to join this platform and to participate in my local MeetUp. This series of groups went on to form what in 2009 would become the anti-establishment Five Star Movement (5SM), one of the two parties forming the current Italian government.

In that national MeetUp forum, in February 2006 a user started a thread called 'Dr Hamer and New Medicine: a shame to keep it hidden from the whole world' (MeetUp 2006a). The first post was a copy of a letter from Mark Pfister, at the time Hamer's right-hand man in Italy and president of the Association of Applied Biological Laws (ALBA), of which Hamer himself was honorary president. Founded in 2003, ALBA gathered more than two thousand supporters in its first year (Marisaldi 2004)—including medical doctors—and organised seminars, conferences, and a 'second opinion' service for patients. In this letter, Mr Pfister incited people to resist the alleged 'world conspiracy' against Hamer, who at the time was serving a prison sentence in France on counts of fraud and illegal practising of medicine (Court of Appeal of Chambery 2005).

The thread was used by Hamer's Italian followers to spread his ideas and to publicise the activities of ALBA and of similar organisations. This thread was always on the first page of the national MeetUp, pushed there by hundreds of Hamer's followers who were enthusiastically encouraging each other, as well as vulnerable people with serious diseases, to abandon science-based treatments in favour of Hamer's theory. For instance, on 20 September 2006 a user, who went by the pseudonym 'Alì Babà', writes:

> For a few weeks I have been feeling a mass, like a lump, on my stomach, but it does not hurt me. I am convinced that it is a tumour, also because thinking about it I discovered the 'biological conflict' that caused it, but I am not afraid because after reading Hamer I know it is not dangerous, and that it will be resolved when I resolve the conflict, so I do not give it so much weight and I almost do not care. And I am also sure that I will not go to any medical doctor to get my examinations and other things, and that I will recover very well without medicines, chemo, radiotherapy or surgery!
> (MeetUp 2006b)

Alì Babà intervenes in the online discussions praising Hamer's theories which, according to him, were even able to 'cure' a child from her Down's syndrome. He is convinced that Hamer's theories 'are simpler and more linear than those of the official medicine, therefore they must surely be truer' (MeetUp 2006b). At the same time, he desperately asks for more information about the cases of a man with a liver tumour, and of a woman with a brain tumour, which were debated in the MeetUp as evidence of the validity of Hamer's theories. He will never receive an answer.

On 29 January 2007, another user posted a letter received from a friend of Alì Babà, describing the latter as a 31-year-old man affected by a particular type of polyposis of the colon, and revealing that he died just before Christmas:

> [He] died suffering in an unspeakable, inhuman way. Until the very last [moment], he refused all treatment and hospitalisation. . ., every drug, even painkillers. He was convinced that goodwill and faith in Hamer would have saved him . . . Unfortunately, it was not so, and his last days were harrowing, he suffered so much! Only now I begin to overcome this tragedy, but the images of his atrocious sufferings will never abandon me!
>
> (*Psiram.com* 2010)

Alì Babà's blind trust in GNM was not an isolated case. In the same forum of MeetUp, the user 'Leonida' wrote that diseases occurring in the Chernobyl area after the infamous disaster were not caused by the radiation but because of 'nostalgia, because the explosion of the power station forced them to move away from the place where they lived' (MeetUp 2007a). Some users were proactively engaging in the dissemination of Hamer's ideas (in line with Lavorgna and Di Ronco 2017). One of ALBA's members, for instance, wrote 'if people would read about Hamer's laws, they could overcome any disease: let's spread them as much as we can' (MeetUp 2006a).

Intrigued by this enthusiasm, I started fact checking these claims: after contacting some German journalists and medical doctors, I discovered that the medical claims in that thread and the story of Hamer's life, as narrated by his followers, were absolutely false. I shared the documents that proved this in the forum, but I was mocked, attacked, and even threatened by Hamer's followers ('you could be an easy target since you are exposing yourself with your real personal data'; 'miserable midge, you are the mud of humanity'). Some users wished me and my family to experience first-hand any form of cancer; others implied I was paid by unspecified pharmaceutical firms to discredit Hamer; others suggested I became a journalist through illegal activities.

About one year after its creation, the thread here discussed reached 322 pages, with more than 186,000 views, and more than 3,200 replies (MeetUp 2007b). After I contacted the MeetUp staff to highlight the public health danger of these discussions, the thread was closed in May 2007, only to reopen two other times (MeetUp 2007c, 2008), when it reached more than 100,000 additional views before being definitively closed.

In an effort to counteract the potential danger of the vast dissemination of this pseudomedicine, both online through MeetUp and offline through the activities of ALBA, I produced an extensive journalistic enquiry for *Cronache del Mezzogiorno* in Salerno, the local newspaper for which I was working at that time. This enquiry, published between April and June 2007, was focused on ALBA and the cases of two people who died following GNM. The enquiry also exposed the fact that one of Hamer's followers was employed by Salerno's main hospital as an X-ray technician in the neuroradiology department, with the risk that these theories may have easily been spread among vulnerable patients. The president of the National Federation for the Orders of Medical Doctors and Dentists (FNOMCeO) acknowledged this risk and promised to look into the issue, but ultimately took no action; the director of the neuroradiology department simply dismissed the risk of exposing his patients to Hamer's theories through the technician. My enquiry was taken up by a colleague of mine who was also working for the national newspaper *Libero*, where he published two articles in September and October 2007 (Rinaldi 2007a, b).

As part of my journalistic efforts, I also helped to write Hamer's entry on the Italian Wikipedia,[1] summarising my findings. This became the centre of an 'edit war' with his followers, who were falsely claiming that the entry did not have a neutral point of view. Subsequently, I was vilified on my Wikipedia user talk page by people stating that I was paid by Big Pharma. I then decided to create the website *Dossier Hamer*,[2] where I published all the documents that I had gathered during my enquiry, including the original copies and the translations of Hamer's trials, and I opened a Facebook page to further spread and discuss my enquiry.[3]

Almost immediately I received abusive comments and emails from Hamer's followers, including legal threats and claims that I was not a 'real' journalist and that my regional Order of Journalists should press charges against me. At the same time, I also received many emails from desperate people who were suffering from serious diseases and, in their frantic search for an answer online, emailed me asking for help in finding a medical doctor who applied the GNM. This shows that even if my website clearly highlighted how Hamer's claims were unsubstantiated and extremely dangerous, potential followers of Hamer, who came across my website, did not necessarily engage with its content. Without reading anything that I had posted, they wrote to me seeking my help in finding a doctor that used Hamer's theories. For example, in May 2008, a 42-year-old woman suffering from multiple myeloma wrote me that she had booked an appointment with Mr Pfister, and wanted more information from me about him. When I invited her to think twice before entrusting her life in the hands of 'therapists' who have never proven their claims, she became furious: she pointed out that she had a master's degree, that her husband was a medical doctor, and that Hamer's and Pfister's theories had indeed been suggested to her by her husband's colleagues. Others sent me their full clinical stories, desperately asking me to pass this information onto Hamer himself or one of the medical doctors who followed him; many others simply wanted to express their disgust for 'official medicine' because it had not been able to cure someone they loved, ultimately venting what they perceived as a betrayal by science-based medicine. However, I also received some encouraging compliments for my work and requests for help from relatives of patients who were following Hamer's theories.

In addition to my efforts to educate the public, I also wrote several emails to local and national FNOMCeO representatives to highlight the dangers of GNM. However, they took no action, and nothing changed from 2007 to 2011. As part of my research into the impact of Hamer's theories in Europe, I got in touch with Nathalie de Reuck, a Belgian journalist who had written a book about how her own mother had died of cancer after following the advice of therapists heavily inspired by Hamer. In January 2011, she interviewed me for the documentary *La médecine qui tue!* (transl. 'The medicine that kills') as part of the programme *Devoir d'enquête* on the public broadcasting TV for the French-speaking Community of Belgium (*RTBF* 2011).

2011–2012: getting national exposure

In April 2011 Domenico Scilipoti, a gynaecologist and acupuncturist who was at the time a member of the Italian Parliament, ran a conference entitled 'The holistic approach to disease and health' (MRNonline.it 2011). Among others, he invited Danilo Toneguzzi to talk about the five Biological Laws discovered by Dr Hamer. Toneguzzi, a psychiatrist and ALBA's president of the scientific committee, at the time was under investigation for the death of his patient Manuela Trevisan, whose story I had followed closely thanks to her mother and friends. In April 2007, Manuela was diagnosed with a non-Hodgkin lymphoma: the hospital's doctor wrote in her medical report that, given the stage and the seriousness of her condition, starting chemotherapy immediately would have given her the only concrete chances of healing. But Manuela was frightened by the chemo, therefore she took some time to think about it; during these days, she learned about Hamer on the internet and discovered that near her hometown there was a medical doctor who was a follower of his theories—that is, the psychiatrist Toneguzzi. Manuela refused any form of science-based treatment and a few months later she wrote in her diary that according to Toneguzzi she could consider herself healed. Five months after writing this, she died. Manuela's family took Toneguzzi to court.

In May 2011, as a consequence of my enquiry, I was invited by the Italian national public broadcasting television company to feature on the popular programme *Mi Manda RaiTre* (a consumer rights programme unmasking scams) in order to expose the dangers of GNM. The television host invited both Scilipoti and Toneguzzi to discuss their views, but the latter elected to send two other members of ALBA in his place. During the programme, Scilipoti fiercely refused to answer why he had given Hamer's theories such a prominent platform at his conference (Ruccia 2011). Following the broadcast, he told Manuela's family that he wanted to help them; but Manuela's mother turned to me for help. Soon after the programme, I drafted a parliamentary question (an instrument of parliamentary oversight in the Italian political system whereby MPs ask the government for information of a factual nature, on behalf of members of the public) for Scilipoti on Hamer's theory and his followers, asking the Health Minister to take a stance against this pseudomedicine. Scilipoti, as a Member of Parliament, officially submitted my question to the Ministry on 23 May 2011 (Camera.it 2011). In March 2012, the Press Office of the Ministry of Health assured me that an answer was imminent. To date, however, my parliamentary question remains unanswered. In 2012, moreover, Toneguzzi was cleared of all charges after a controversial trial in which the judge came to the conclusion that Toneguzzi had used Hamer's theories only for making diagnoses and not for actually attempting to cure patients (Court Trial of Pordenone 2012). Even after the TV programme, therefore, nothing had changed: amid the indifference of the public and the authorities, Hamer's followers continued to claim they were persecuted while organising seminars, selling books, and applying the GNM to many vulnerable individuals.

2016-current: the renewed media attention, and recent and continuing dissemination activities

It was only in 2016, when a series of people died after following GNM, that Hamer's ideas fell once again under the media's spotlight. Among the cases which reached media attention are those of Cristian Trevisan, a 35-year-old lorry driver with a Hodgkin lymphoma (Nicolussi Moro 2017) who was under the care of the family doctor Paolo Rossaro, who was subsequently expelled from the FNOMCeO; Alessandra Tosi, a 34-year-old mother of two with breast cancer, who died after 'curing' it with compresses of ricotta and nettles (*Corriere.it* 2016) (this case, however, is controversial because there is no clear proof that she was following Hamer's theories since the onset of her cancer); Marina Lallo, a 53-year-old woman who let her small and treatable melanoma grow until it metastasised all over her body and killed her (Martinenghi 2018); and Eleonora Bottaro, whose parents were vocal Hamer followers. Eleonora was only 17 years old when diagnosed with a form of leukaemia that is highly curable with chemotherapy; however, she refused any science-based treatment and died a few days after her 18th birthday.

Because of this renewed interest in Hamer's theories in the media, in September 2016 I was interviewed by the Italian edition of the magazine *Vanity Fair* (Nucini 2016), where I recounted the details of my enquiry and questioned why authorities—in particular the FNOMCeO and the National Agency for Regional Health Services—did not intervene to address this issue. As I documented, some of Hamer's followers had even been able to host courses that were accredited for Continuing Medical Education credits, which each professional in the health sector must acquire every year. Additionally, between 2015 and 2017, a medical doctor claimed he taught several courses of 'holistic gynaecology' using Hamer's theories and books as part of the academic programme at the University of Salerno (D'Amato 2017a). I alerted the local FNOMCeO board and the university, but neither of them replied to my letters. In January 2017, I had the chance to discuss my enquiry during the public television programme *PresaDiretta* (which focuses on cases of investigative journalism), which broadcasted a special episode on health charlatans, featuring also a long segment on Hamer's theories (*PresaDiretta* 2017). In April that year, the Italian-speaking public Swiss TV company broadcasted a segment entitled 'Cancer, the false promise' focusing on some of Hamer's Italian victims and on Mark Pfister, who was still practising as a 'therapist' in Switzerland (Bernasconi 2017). In this segment, a journalist pretended to be affected by a malignant squamous cell carcinoma in her cervix (with metastases that could have been treated with both radiotherapy and chemotherapy). During the appointment, Pfister reiterated Hamer's idea that metastasis do not exist and that her cancer was just a scar, caused by the 'biological conflict' of her sexual dissatisfaction; he also suggested that she delayed her treatment until she was visited by an Italian gynaecologist chosen by him. Despite the public attention reached through these television programmes, once again public authorities took no action.

In the meantime, I was able to successfully pitch my journalistic enquiry to the major Italian publisher Mondadori, and in 2017, 10 years after the start of my enquiry, I finally published the book *Dossier Hamer* (D'Amato 2017b). The book quickly gained visibility in national media (Remuzzi 2017), especially after Hamer's death in July 2017 (Bianchi 2017; Longo 2017). In nine months, *Dossier Hamer* sold about 1,600 copies: all the profit I gained from it was donated to Cancer Research UK and Macmillan Cancer Support in equal parts.

Among other things, I also took part in the panel 'Health's mythology and false arguments: the hoaxes' era' organised by the FNOMCeO (2017) as part of the Festival of TV and New Media in Piedmont. The panel, where renowned journalists and medical doctors debated the best strategy to counteract the dangers of so-called medical fake news, signalled a recognition from the medical board of my own work: for the first time, the board listened to the concerns expressed in my enquiry. The different attitude of the FNOMCeO towards hoaxes in the medical arena is also confirmed by a civil action that was brought against a physician follower of Hamer's theories by the board's Turin section a few months before our meeting. The court case resulted in the conviction of the physician, who was found liable for the manslaughter of Marina Lallo (*La Repubblica* 2016).

After the launch of the book, I redesigned my website and have added a blog, which I have used alongside the dedicated Facebook page, to better update my audience on the developments that occurred after the book's printing. My intended audience is people who are thinking about using GNM to 'cure' themselves because they are too scared of science-based treatments. However, once again, Hamer's followers used these new media (the blog and the Facebook page) to reiterate lies about Hamer's life, vent the perceived danger and corruption of the medical system, and wish me cancer. I have always tried to adopt a firm but calm tone, even against the more disrespectful users—with whom I try to engage; the only behaviour that I have not tolerated on my pages is the spamming of unsubstantiated claims and personal insults against other users and victims of Hamer's theories. Those who behave in this way are banned.

Despite my efforts, throughout the last 10 years my work has reached a limited audience. More recently, however, my work has gained a wider audience through the references that some visible scientists/doctors—such as Salvo Di Grazia (gynaecologist and debunker) and Roberto Burioni (professor of microbiology and virology, and active campaigner against anti-vaccination activists, see also Chapter 9)—have made to it (Medbunker 2017; Burioni 2018).

Factual debunking in a polarised world

My experience taught me that factual debunking alone is not enough to change the minds of the followers of dangerous pseudo-medicines. I have written about Hamer for over 10 years, trying to disseminate the results of my enquiries as broadly as I could. Nonetheless, the popularity of GNM continues to grow, with new practitioners coming to light all the time. I constantly receive emails and tips about GNM practitioners operating in Italy; unfortunately, I do not have the time and the means to follow up on all these clues by embarking on complex journalistic enquiries, writing blogs, and alerting the relevant medical associations of the dangerous nonmedical practices adopted by some of their members.

The fact that GNM retains its popularity might lead us to conclude that investigative journalism alone (and its efforts to present to the public accurate facts) seems to be unsustainable and relatively ineffective: my enquiry about Hamer was something that I undertook on top of my daily work commitments; I self-funded the translations of legal documents (that formed the core of my enquiry) and the hosting of my website; my enquiry also placed a strain on me from an emotional point of view, as I had to interview many people who were describing the dreadful suffering of their beloved friends or relatives. Many interviews ended with me shedding tears after hanging up the phone, and to date these stories still haunt me. What kept me going—and tolerating the insults, threats, and the silence of the authorities who should have protected the victims of Hamer's circle—was the conviction that my efforts helped my audience to make informed choices about their health care (with potential life-saving results).

It is worth noting that I am not the only journalist who has written on Hamer. A number of investigative journalists across Europe have highlighted the damage caused by GNM over time. A case that received extensive media coverage by all main European media, for instance, is that of Olivia Pilhar, a six-year-old Austrian who in 1995 was diagnosed with a malignant kidney tumour and was forced by her parents to leave the hospital and follow Hamer's treatments in Spain. After the intervention of the Austrian state, Olivia was brought back to the hospital and saved, while her parents were sentenced to eight months' probation for negligent assault and deprivation of a minor from the power of the guardian (*Die Presse* 2010). Despite the media coverage, however, Hamer's ideas continued to gain momentum in Europe and particularly in Italy. Olivia's parents have given lectures and organised seminars promoting

GNM, and sold books about their story.[4] This raises the question of why the public fails to hear (or does not want to hear) our warnings.

Research suggests that, when confronted with events we cannot completely understand but which deeply affect our lives, we tend to face them using our own 'narrative' (Quattrociocchi and Vicini 2016). When antagonised by a conflicting narrative, our confirmation bias will selectively filter only the information that fits our own narrative. In the case illustrated in this chapter, this means that all documents and scientific evidence about the dangers of Hamer's theory will simply be ignored by his followers. This phenomenon is particularly evident online, where opposing groups fight without really listening to each other and discourses become easily polarised (Del Vicario 2016a; see Chapter 9 of this book).

This problem is worsened by the fact that many of Hamer's followers discuss their health issues in closed digital groups. In this way, they can better protect their narrative and the medical doctors who practice GNM (in line with Lavorgna and Di Ronco 2017). Taking refuge on social media causes a 'shift of paradigm in the creation and consumption of information', where:

> We passed from a mediated (e.g., by journalists) to a more disintermediated selection process. Such a disintermediation elicits the tendencies of the users to a) select information adhering to their system of beliefs—i.e., confirmation bias—and b) to form groups of like-minded people where they polarize their opinion—i.e. echo chamber.
>
> (Del Vicario 2016b:1)

Additionally, Hamer's victims are often kept isolated from their families, in a sect-like environment (D'Amato 2017b). This isolation is also a by-product of what Kahan (2017) defines as 'identity protective cognition', which can be defined as 'the tendency of culturally diverse individuals to selectively credit and dismiss evidence in patterns that reflect the beliefs that predominate in their group' (Kahan 2017:1). In essence, this means that members of GNM groups would tend to dismiss every health-related recommendation that threatens the values of their group (e.g., to undergo chemo or visit a hospital), even if it comes from their own relatives.

Because of the limitations of factual debunking and the difficulties in breaking into online echo chambers, in *Dossier Hamer*, my book, I have tried to strike a balance between underlining the dangers of Hamer's pseudomedicine and showing compassion for the victims. In this way, I could reach those scared by science-based medicine and its treatments who were considering trying the GNM themselves, or suggest it to their loved ones, and had genuine doubts about what to do. Despite being constantly guided by journalistic rigour, I used a storytelling approach that aimed at giving voice to the victims (whose emotions and experiences were reconstructed mostly through their families' accounts and extensive documentation). In addition, I also established a close relationship with those who told me their stories: for instance, the mother of

Manuela Trevisan (see previous). She did not attend the court trials regarding her daughter's death—the pain was simply too much; and yet, she had the courage to appear on national TV to tell her daughter's story on the condition that I was by her side.

Complicating the narratives

Understanding what investigative and scientific journalism could (or should) do to expose dangerous forms of pseudomedicine without becoming 'activism' is not a simple matter. Indeed, the journalistic practice of simply presenting data to the public is not effective, nor is trying to 'debunk' or to ridicule pseudo-scientific narratives, which in some cases are deeply embedded in the way some people frame the world. An alternative approach is therefore needed.

Some years ago, the predominant approach in the public communication of science was the 'information deficit model' (Bodmer 1985), which assumes that the public's distrust of science comes from a lack of accurate information. Many lack sufficient knowledge about science (which is why many of them distrust it), and should therefore be properly educated by scientists. This top-down approach presents science as a monolithic entity where the experts pour specialist knowledge into an undifferentiated, and ignorant, general public. It has also proven quite ineffective. Indeed, when journalists try to counteract scientific misinformation simply by debunking, they can actually increase the proliferation and the strength of that misinformation—this is the so-called backfire effect (Peter and Koch 2016). Today we know that a more efficient approach is to 'empower' the public through a bi-directional process (Gregory and Lock 2008): this is particularly urgent in Italy, where mainstream media treat scientific communication as a 'battlefield', particularly around the no- vs pro-vax issue (Villa 2019; see chapters 6 and 9).

Given this context, what is the role of journalism and journalists in counteracting the spread of scientific misinformation? When it comes to health-related news, correct information can literally make the difference between the life and death of people (misinforming them may lead them to undergo non-science-based practices); at the same time, it would be presumptuous for journalists, and inevitably frustrating for them, to aim at eradicating all medical misinformation and charlatans. However, in exposing quack doctors, my experience taught me that there is also an additional layer of difficulty in the slowness and the corporatism of many medical organisations (such as the FNOMCeO in Italy) in tackling their members' mistakes. For years, I have contacted all the relevant authorities to alert them about the dangers of the GNM. However, they have either ignored me or promised actions that never followed. It is only when this issue made the headlines of national newspapers that I was taken seriously by the FNOMCeO. Still, my enquiry and its follow-ups show that to date there are many medical doctors who, directly or indirectly—but always in a very public way—use Hamer's theories in their daily interactions with their patients. Worth mentioning is the fact that FNOMCeO cannot take action when their members are undergoing trial until the judicial process is completed, to protect themselves from potential litigation in case its members are found innocent at the end of their judicial trial. Since Italian trials are notoriously slow, this means that a medical doctor who adheres to Hamer's theories can continue to practice for many years, even if under trial. For example, Paolo Rossaro's trial started in 2007, but he was only expelled from the board 10 years later. Even the Ministry of Health had been completely unresponsive on this issue.

Hence, a well-informed audience is probably the best way to hold accountable both Hamer's followers and the authorities and to avoid many more victims. To achieve this level of involvement of the public, the lesson for journalists not willing to overstep their role and become activists is, as Amanda Ripley suggests in a recent essay, to 'complicate the narrative' (Ripley 2017). As I have tried to do with my enquiry, it is important to understand people's motivations: in particular, we should try to listen more extensively and closely, and to use the language of care. These are certainly great starting points to lower polarisation in the public discourse, especially in the algorithm-driven social media debate. My own experience in debating Hamer's theories with his followers on social media suggests that often these people just want to express frustration towards a medical environment that they perceive as impersonal, sterile, and personally damaging. It is not rare for cancer patients, cured with science-based treatments, to feel that the GNM would have been a better option for them. Too often, they fear that invasive science-based treatments are not balanced by their positive outcomes. Pointing out statistics or insisting on logical contradictions would not create any dialogue, but only further conflict.

Therefore, I have chosen an approach that takes into account this irrational but very real fear. By using Ripley's 'language of care', I try to display from the very beginning my sincere empathy towards someone who has to face terrible diagnoses and treatments with awful side effects. In addition, I try to build a bridge between me and these scared people, making it clear that we both want the same things: a medicine that cures as many people as possible, but also a medicine which is more humane and understandable and free from economic and political motives. The problem is that both sides think 'their truth' is 'the Truth': it is only by breaking the bubble and building a bridge based on understanding the others' viewpoints that we, as journalists, can make the first step towards showing science for what it is, not what we want it to be.

The already mentioned work by Quattrociocchi and Vicini (2016) is crucial to understanding the real extent of polarisation on social media, and how a certain type of 'aggressive debunking' is not only useless as a tool for changing society's attitude towards science, but can even become harmful for the public debate. Unfortunately, the latest report from the Italian Authority for Communications Guarantees shows that even if 56% of the public is 'very or extremely interested' in science and technology, 'specialist topics are often treated by journalists who do not have a specific basic preparation' (*AGCOM* 2018:22; see Chapter 11). These non-specialist journalists promote an over-simplified version of science—particularly medical science—in order to appeal to an audience that desperately needs to divide the world into two clear camps, transforming the scientific debate into a highly divisive politicised topic (Sandal 2019).

Some people perceive medical science as an anti-democratic entity that makes important decisions about their bodies and the bodies of their loved ones. In addition, science is also perceived by many as something 'magic' because of its rapid development in recent years, which has not yet been culturally 'absorbed' by society. All these reasons may push at least some people to turn towards pseudomedicine promising even more 'magic' solutions, such as the GNM. It is therefore necessary to work on making science more accessible, because 'communications can't fix a problem you don't understand' (Larson 2014:84). The approach suggested by Ripley (2017), to use the language of care, can be a good starting point for bridging the gap of trust between the scientific community and the general public—a gap that journalists can also help to fill. Of course, this cannot be considered a magic formula to be applied across the board by anyone and to every audience. Complexity (including in medical discoveries and health practices) can be scary for the public. Exposing ourselves and our readers to the nuances of the issues we tackle is the only way to start piercing the echo chamber we live in, both online and offline.

Conclusion

This chapter shows how medical misinformation is a pressing issue in the public debate. Journalism has not yet found a unique solution to counteract it, but from literature and experience we know what does not work: polarisation and engagement only within isolated echo chambers. My experience with the GNM and the misinformation spread by Hamer's followers indicates that simply presenting documents in a transparent, traceable way does nothing to counteract the false claims of these followers in their own echo chambers (in line with Del Vicario 2016a,b). However, with *Dossier Hamer*, I have adopted a blended approach using non-fictional elements to humanise the stories of the GNM's victims, trying to appeal to a set of basic human emotions shared by everyone. This approach, which values the personal story behind the misunderstanding of how medicine works, coupled with a constant explanation of the basic mechanisms of science, tries to appeal to those who are scared of science-based treatments but have not yet formed a definitive opinion about Hamer's theories. It might not be possible to draw any definitive conclusion about the effectiveness of such an approach. However, we know that an aggressive, top-down style of communication about science is not only problematic but probably also ineffective (Villa 2019). Journalists can and must play a bigger role in the public debate about medical miscommunication, not only by undertaking more specialised training in scientific fields, but also by embracing a more open, transparent, and especially empathic approach to science communication.

Notes

1 See it.wikipedia.org/wiki/Ryke_Geerd_Hamer.
2 See www.dossierhamer.it.
3 www.facebook.com/DossierHamer.
4 See www.germanische-heilkunde.at.

References

Administrative Court of Frankfurt Am Main (2003) Dr. med. Ryke Geerd Hamer vs State of Hesse, case 12 E 591/03 (2). Available at: www.dossierhamer.it/wp-content/uploads/2017/03/VF12E59103.pdf

AGCOM (2018) News vs. fake nel sistema dell'informazione. Available at: www.agcom.it/documents/10179/3744102/Allegato+22-11-2018/3aff8790-8039-4456-8f9a-dae2497289a4

Bernasconi A (2017) *Cancro, le false promesse*. Radiotelevisione svizzera di lingua italiana. Apr 6. Available at: www.rsi.ch/la1/programmi/informazione/falo/tutti-i-servizi/Il-cancro-non-fa-male-8954062.html

Bianchi L (2017) Il giornalista italiano che da dieci anni documenta la follia della Nuova Medicina Germanica. *Vice*. Jul 11. Available at: www.vice.com/it/article/a3dk5p/nuova-medicina-germanica-ilario-damato-hamer

Bodmer W (1985) *The public understanding of science*. London: Royal Society

Burioni R (2018) *Balle mortali*. Milan: Rizzoli

Camera.it (2011) Interrogazione a risposta scritta 4–12035. Available at: http://banchedati.camera.it/sindacatoispettivo_16/showXhtml.Asp?idAtto=39267&stile=6&highLight=1

Camilletti F (2007) Interview with Dr. Hamer. Sept 23. Available at: https://web.archive.org/web/20160304063904/www.nuovamedicinagermanica.it/index.php?option=com_content&task=view&id=98&Itemid=41

Corriere.it (2016) Rifiuta cure per metodo Hamer, un'altra donna morta a Rimini. Sept 3. Available at: www.corriere.it/cronache/16_settembre_03/rifiuta-cure-metodo-hamer-donna-morta-rimini-a477c27c-71af-11e6-a5ab-6335286216cb.shtml

Court of Appeal of Chambery (2005) FB/EC Dossier no. 02/00261, arret no. 04/515. Available at: www.dossierhamer.it/blog/portfolio/chambery04/

Court Trial of Pordenone (2012) trial 11 January 2012, reference n. 3394/08 R.G. N.R., n. 831/09 R.G. Trib., n. 5/12 Reg. Sent

D'Amato I (2017a) Hamer all'Università di Salerno? *Dossier Hamer Blog*. Available at: www.dossierhamer.it/blog/hamer-universita-salerno/

D'Amato I (2017b) *Dossier Hamer*. Milano: Mondadori

Deckers, A (2008) List of known victims. Available at: www.ariplex.com/ama/ama_ham2.htm

Del Vicario M, Bessi A, Zollo F, Petroni F, Scala A and Caldarelli G et al. (2016a) The spreading of misinformation online. *Proceedings of The National Academy of Sciences* 113(3):554–559

Del Vicario M, Vivaldo G, Bessi A, Zollo F, Scala A, Caldarelli G and Quattrociocchi W. (2016b). Echo chambers: emotional contagion and group polarization on Facebook. *Scientific Reports* 6:37825

Die Presse (2010) Victim and media star: the case of Olivia Pilhar. *Panorama*. Available at: https://diepresse.com/home/panorama/oesterreich/533340/Opfer-und-Medienstar_Der-Fall-Olivia-Pilha

Gregory J and Lock SJ (2008) The evolution of 'public understanding of science': public engagement as a tool of science policy in the UK. *Sociology Compass* 2:1252–1265

Grillo B (2005) *Incontriamoci: meetup*. Available at: www.beppegrillo.it/incontriamoci-meetup/

FNOMCeO (2017) *La Fnomceo a Dogliani contro le fake news in medicina*. Available at: https://portale.fnomceo.it/wp-content/uploads/2017/11/La_Professione_1-2017._Mitologia_della_salute_e_false_argomentazioni_Dogliani_.pdf

Hamer RG (2005) *The five biological laws of the new medicine*. Amici di Dirk, Ediciones de la Nueva Medicina SL. Available at: www.germannewmedicine.ca/documents/Madrid-2005-en.PDF

Hamer RG (2010) *Open letter*. Germanic-new-medicine.com. Available at: https://web.archive.org/web/20110815053742/http://dr-rykegeerdhamer.com/index.php?option=com_content&task=view&id=362&Itemid=76

Kahan Dan M (2017) *Misconceptions, misinformation, and the logic of identity-protective cognition*. Cultural Cognition Project Working Paper Series No. 164. Yale Law School, Public Law Research Paper No. 605; Yale Law & Economics Research Paper No. 575

La Repubblica (2017) Torino, cura-beffa anticancro: l'Ordine dei medici si costituirà parte civile contro l'omeopata. Apr 22, 2016. Available at: https://torino.repubblica.it/cronaca/2016/04/22/news/torino_cura-beffa_anticancro_l_ordine_dei_medici_si_costituira_parte_civile_contro_l_omeopata-138241153/

Larson H (2014) Underlying issues are key to dispelling vaccine doubts. *Bulletin of the World Health Organization* (92):84–85

Lavorgna A and Di Ronco A (2017) Fraud victims or unwary accomplices? An exploratory study of online communities supporting quack medicine. In Van Duyne PC, Harvey J, Antonopoulos GA and Von Lampe K (eds.) *The many faces of crime for profit and ways of tackling it*. Nijmegen, NL: Wolf Legal Publishers

Lofstad R (2017) Controversial German 'doctor' who was resident in Sandefjord is dead. *Dagbladet*. Jul 5. Available at: www.dagbladet.no/nyheter/omstridt-tysk-lege-bosatt-i-sandefjord-er-dod/68470613

Longo AR (2017) Metodo Hamer: una nuova intervista a Ilario D'Amato. *Query*. Oct 3. Available at: www.queryonline.it/2017/10/03/metodo-hamer-una-nuova-intervista-a-ilario-damato/

Marisaldi G (2004) Letter to Amnesty International 21 October 2004. Available at: http://free-news.org/hamer37.htm

Martinenghi S (2018) Torino, condanna inasprita in appello per la dottoressa che curò un melanoma con l'omeopatia. *Repubblica.it*. Oct 26. Available at: https://torino.repubblica.it/cronaca/2018/10/26/news/torino_condanna_inasprita_in_appello_per_la_dottoressa_che_curo_un_melanoma_con_l_omeopatia-210064916/

MedBunker (2017) Facebook post. Jul 26. Available at: www.facebook.com/MedBunker/photos/a.311358395559438/1735202269841703

MeetUp.com (2006a) Available at: https://web.archive.org/web/20061009200532/http://beppegrillo.meetup.com:80/boards/view/viewthread?thread=1671117

MeetUp.com (2006b) Available at: https://web.archive.org/web/20090116213657/http://beppegrillo.meetup.com/boards/thread/1671117/160/

MeetUp.com (2007a) Available at: https://web.archive.org/web/20081214162725/http://beppegrillo.meetup.com/boards/thread/1671117/1950/

MeetUp.com (2007b) Available at: https://web.archive.org/web/20070509210448/http://beppegrillo.meetup.com:80/boards/

MeetUp.com (2007c) Available at: https://web.archive.org/web/20080118151641/http://beppegrillo.meetup.com:80/boards/

MeetUp.com (2008) Available at: https://web.archive.org/web/20080228211913/http://beppegrillo.meetup.com:80/boards/

MRNonline.it (2011) Available at: https://web.archive.org/web/20110415191758/www.mrnonline.it/?p=402

Nicolussi Moro M (2017) Niente chemio per curare il linfoma, l'Ordine radia medico di famiglia. *Il Corriere del Veneto*. Jun 14. Available at: https://corrieredelveneto.corriere.it/veneziamestre/notizie/cronaca/2017/14-giugno-2017/niente-chemio-curare-linfoma-l-ordine-radia-medico-famiglia-2401681732725.shtml

Nucini S (2016) Metodo Hamer: sveglia, dottori! *Vanity Fair*. Sept 15. Available at: www.vanityfair.it/news/storie/16/09/15/metodo-hamer-storia

Peter C and Koch T (2016) When debunking scientific myths fails (and when it does not): the backfire effect in the context of journalistic coverage and immediate judgments as prevention strategy. *Science Communication* 38(1):3–25

PresaDiretta (2017) Ciarlatani. Jan 16. Available at: www.presadiretta.rai.it/dl/portali/site/puntata/ContentItem-aed935af-e750-418b-8618-c23e3c175990.html

Psiram.com (2010) *Caso Aldo*. Available at: www.psiram.com/it/index.php/Caso_Aldo

Quattrociocchi W and Vicini A (2016) *Misinformation*. Milano: Franco Angeli

Remuzzi G (2017) Hamer spacciatore di falsi prodigi. Il ghiaccio come cura dei tumori. *Corriere della Sera*. Mar 28. Available at: www.corriere.it/cultura/17_marzo_27/dossier-hamer-d-amato-libro-4886194a-131d-11e7-be9a-6ca09ed8307d.shtml

Rinaldi P (2007a) Il pensiero cura il tumore, l'ultima truffa new age. *Libero*. Sept 25, p. 21

Rinaldi P (2007b) Il ministero boccia la setta-anticancro. *Libero*. Oct 14, p. 21

Ripley A (2017) Complicating the narratives. *The Whole Story*. Available at: https://thewholestory.solutionsjournalism.org/complicating-the-narratives-b91ea06ddf63

RTBF (2011) La médecine qui tue! *Devoir d'enquête*. Jan 12, Radio-Télévision belge de la Fédération Wallonie-Bruxelles

Ruccia G (2011) Scilipoti-show a 'Mi manda Raitre'. *IlFattoQuotidiano.it*. Available at: https://web.archive.org/web/20110713155408/www.ilfattoquotidiano.it/2011/05/07/scilipoti-show-a-mi-manda-raitre/109642/

Sandal M (2019) Scienza e potere. *Esquire*. Jan 11. Available at: www.esquire.com/it/news/attualita/a25843918/vaccini-scienza-democratica/

Sigmaringen's Administrative Court (2005) Urteil vom 09.06.2005–8 K 610/03. Available at: https://openjur.de/u/607476.html

Villa R (2019) La comunicazione della scienza non è un campo di battaglia. *Wired*. Jan 15. Available at: www.wired.it/scienza/medicina/2019/01/15/comunicazione-scienza-burioni/

13 Concluding thoughts

Anita Lavorgna and Anna Di Ronco

Getting to grips with non-science-based health practices

With this edited volume, we aimed to provide a platform to engage with the issue of medical misinformation by using a diverse range of empirical and theoretical insights from different disciplines, including criminology, digital sociology, health psychology, medicine, law, physics, and journalism. Our multidisciplinary approach allowed us to bring together researchers and even practitioners from a variety of different background who had the possibility to draw on their own specialties and capitalise on their expertise in order to head towards a common direction—the tackling of harmful non-science-based health practices and the misinformation surrounding them. We hope that our readers will benefit from being exposed to ideas and knowledge otherwise unusual to them—a perk of multidisciplinarity.

At the beginning of this edited book we began by clarifying that under the umbrella of non-science-based health practices a plethora of distinct behaviours causing social or even criminal harm can be found; these behaviours can often be passively accepted, approved, or even commended by people because of the misinformation surrounding them. Not all non-science-based health practices are, however, necessarily harmful. For this reason, we have stressed the importance of being respectful of the context-specific character of many alternative health practices, whose definitions, perceptions, and responses are very much shaped by their socio-cultural and even historical background. Of course, being attentive to the way alternative and non-science-based health practices are understood and regulated, especially in western societies, does not mean that they should be uncritically accepted—especially if they are biologically implausible, fraudulent, or variously harmful to both individuals and society. There is a thin line between healing approaches that are valued in certain cultural traditions, those acceptable within the boundaries of (informed) patient choice in healthcare (which are usually harmless), and those that should be somehow disapproved, condemned, or even prohibited because of their dangerousness. Even if the line between these behaviours is a thin one, a line nevertheless exists. We carefully pondered on where to draw this line in this book: this task was at times very easy, and at times necessarily tentative. Nonetheless, we believe that reflecting on the positioning of this line is not a futile exercise, but rather a necessary one to advance debates on alternative and integrative health practices.

This line positioning exercise, however, is often overlooked. Public debates tend to be much polarised, with people considering both harmful and harmless alternative practices either as acceptable or as entirely unacceptable. Polarisation also makes it hard for state regulators to approach non-science-based medical practices and their boundaries. In practice, this means that it may be difficult for them to address a number of questions, including how much should the state validate or even subsidise non-science-based integrative medicine? On which basis and how much (if at all) should it limit individuals' self-determination in healthcare, including their freedom to choose health treatments for their children? Answering these questions has become increasingly hard for the state, and for intellectuals and social and medical scientists within it, especially given the increasing popularity of some alternative health practices (and the online misinformation supporting their use). Perhaps we should come to terms with the fact that, at least when it comes to non-science-based health practices, a full and complete reconciliation among 'sceptics' and 'believers' might never occur—after all, healthcare choices can be deeply personal and relate to individuals' philosophical views on individual freedom and social responsibility. Nonetheless, we believe that it is of the upmost importance to reduce the epistemological gap between these two factions by providing a more scientifically informed (yet context-sensitive) understanding of the effectiveness and the potential harms of specific non-science-based pharmaceuticals and treatments.

So, how can we further improve our understanding of non-science-based health practices, the social harms they can cause, and the mechanisms of misinformation surrounding them?

In current times of crisis of public trust in expert knowledge (including biomedical) and of widespread misinformation, new efforts are needed by research communities to better understand harmful non-science-based health practices. In particular, research communities need to better grasp their causes, characteristics, and impact, as well as the way in which they successfully build support and propagate findings online and offline. Of course, scientific endeavours are especially needed to identify the best ways to address *harmful* non-science-based health practices and reduce their negative impact on society. This is why we strongly believe that further studies, including of a comparative nature, need to be conducted in the area, and that many more disciplines, including and beyond the ones in this book, need to engage with this inherently multifaceted and complex problem. For this edited book, we invited authors from criminology, digital sociology, health psychology, medicine, law, physics, and journalism to contribute with a chapter. Of course, we are aware that this is only a starting point: many more disciplines—including health humanities, economics, and ethics—are likely to have a lot to say to further research in this topic.

This book mostly relied on a multidisciplinary approach. This means that it has drawn on intellectual and methodological insights from different disciplines, which have mainly worked independently one alongside each other. Multidisciplinarity is an important prerequisite to trans- and interdisciplinary, which, we believe, should be the next logical steps to be taken in the effort to tackle the many problems surrounding non-science-based medical approaches. *Transdiciplinarity*, in particular, is the approach that would allow social, natural, and health scientists to tackle common problems by transcending their traditional disciplinary boundaries and, therefore, by integrating their knowledge and methodological approaches. In the ideally next logical step, *interdisciplinarity* would allow researchers to harmonise and synthesise all their different disciplinary approaches into a coherent whole, thus refining and enhancing societal understandings of harmful non-science-based practices. Of course, trans- and interdisciplinarity approaches are complex, as they require different disciplines and professions to make a serious effort in understanding each other's language, theoretical and methodological frameworks, and standards—which may vary considerably across them. Some of the chapters in this volume attempted trans- and interdisciplinarity approaches and we hope they can lay the ground for new efforts in this direction.

We must acknowledge, however, that trans- and interdisciplinarity approaches suffer from a very practical problem: the relative absence of incentives to carry out trans- and interdisciplinarity work in academia. Interdisciplinarity studies, indeed, are often difficult to publish (most highly ranked journals are mono-disciplinary) and to 'pigeonhole' for job or funding applications, thus hindering academics' career progression. Difficulties also emerge when work is carried out to bridge the gap between academics and other relevant professionals, ranging from journalists and debunkers to doctors and policy makers. In these cases, it can be complicated for both academics and professionals to initiate a dialogue between one another and to collaborate in joint research or outreach projects—collaboration may often be hindered by the reluctance from both sides to get involved in fields and areas where not only the language and standards, but also the main aims, tend to differ. In the few instances when collaboration between academics and professionals does take place, it can be difficult for academics and professionals alike to capitalise on what they can offer: theoretical and methodological knowledge and rigour, and invaluable on-the-ground experience and understanding. Despite these difficulties, the creation of collaborative communities seems the best way forward—this will certainly help not only to improve our understanding of harmful non-science-based health practices, but also to generate a real societal impact by narrowing the knowing-doing gap and raising public awareness.

A final reminder

This edited book is the tangible result of preliminary and still ongoing efforts to open a dialogue across academic disciplines, and between them and non-academic professionals, on medical misinformation and social harms in non-science-based health practices. The behavioural typologies suggested, the case studies exemplified, and the exploratory analyses presented are all informative starting points from which to learn—also in future comparative studies—and to foster new critical thinking. We approached the editing of this book with a desire to engage in crucial and topical debates surrounding non-science-based health practices and health-related misinformation, being conscious that this is only a beginning of a journey and certainly not the end of it. We hope that this journey will contribute, at least in small part, to increasing awareness, reducing victimisation, and mitigating harms to the past and current victims or unwary supporters of harmful health-related practices.

Index

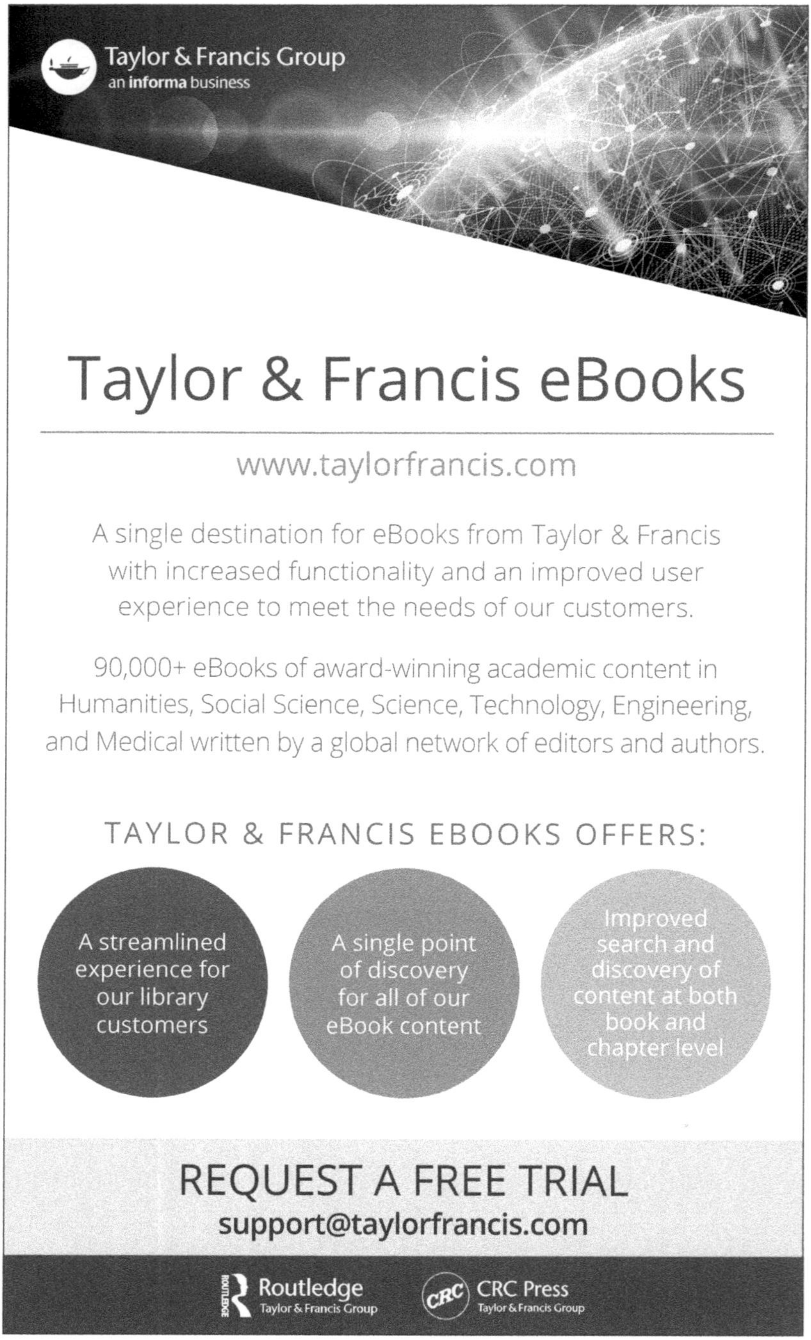
Taylor & Francis Group
an informa business
Taylor & Francis eBooks
www.taylorfrancis.com
A single destination for eBooks from Taylor & Francis with increased functionality and an improved user experience to meet the needs of our customers.
90,000+ eBooks of award-winning academic content in Humanities, Social Science, Science, Technology, Engineering, and Medical written by a global network of editors and authors.
TAYLOR & FRANCIS EBOOKS OFFERS:
A streamlined experience for our library customers
A single point of discovery for all of our eBook content
Improved search and discovery of content at both book and chapter level
REQUEST A FREE TRIAL
support@taylorfrancis.com
Routledge
Taylor & Francis Group
CRC Press
Taylor & Francis Group

www.ingramcontent.com/pod-product-compliance
Ingram Content Group UK Ltd.
Pitfield, Milton Keynes, MK11 3LW, UK
UKHW011013180926
475701UK00004B/716
9781032087535